RECOVERING FROM MILD TRAUMATIC BRAIN INJURY (MTBI)

A Handbook of Hope for Our Military Warriors and Their Families

---

Based on *Mild Traumatic Brain Injury: A Survivor's Handbook*

by Theta Theta No Beta

EDITED BY
MARY ANN KEATLEY, PhD, CCC
AND LAURA L WHITTEMORE

A BRAIN INJURY HOPE FOUNDATION PUBLICATION

Brain Injury Hope Foundation
P. O. Box 1319
Boulder, CO 80306

Telephone: 303-484-2126
www.BrainInjuryHopeFoundation.org

Proceeds from book sales are donated to the Brain Injury Hope Foundation, a nonprofit organization that provides financial assistance to individuals with MTBI. The Foundation's mission is to also promote awareness and understanding of mild traumatic brain injury.

Disclaimer: This book is not designed to replace a physician's independent judgment about the appropriateness or risks of a procedure or therapy for a given patient. Our purpose is to provide you with information and understanding that will help you make confident health care decisions.

Cover design by Tony Greco
www.tonygrecodesign.com

Interior illustrations by Kersti Frigell
kfrigell@comcast.net

Photos by Barbara Colombo
www.11-11productions.com

Interior design, composition and copyediting by Dianne Nelson
Shadow Canyon Graphics
www.shadowcanyongraphics.com

Library of Congress Control Number: 2009931075
ISBN: 978-0-9824094-0-4
Printed in the United States of America

TABLE OF CONTENTS

Definition of MTBI
MTBI Often Goes Unidentified or Misdiagnosed
Definition of Post Traumatic Stress Disorder (PTSD)

Physical Symptoms
Emotional Symptoms
Cognitive or Thinking Symptoms
Effects of Barometric Pressure and Altitude
You Don't Know What You Don't Know

Hearing Problems and Hypersensitivity To Sound
Vision Problems and Sensitivity to Light
Dizziness and Vertigo
Changes in Energy Reserve After Injury

ACKNOWLEDGMENTS

We wish to acknowledge that this book was inspired by a little handbook entitled, *Mild Traumatic Brain Injury: A Survivor's Handbook*, written by Theta Theta No Beta, a Colorado based MTBI support group and edited in 1995 by Robin Murphy Davis. Robin was one of the original authors of the Survivor's Handbook and a beloved member of our community. She was a member of the Brain Trust and an inspiration to all those she touched.

The name Theta Theta No Beta is a reference to brain waves. Those suffering from MTBI often have an increase in theta waves and a decrease in beta waves. Members of Theta Theta No Beta are Leana Bowman, Maurene Flory, Lori Maki, Bhadra Mitchell, Lesley Reed, Connie Scribner, Robin Murphy Davis, Judith Frans, Maria Michael, Laura Phillips, Carol Roberts, and Katy H. Wolf. Their efforts to produce the book were encouraged and supported by Mary Lou Acimovic, MA, CCC-Sp, who contributed expertise and editorial assistance throughout the process; and Jan Lemmon, PhD., who shared her knowledge and scholarly advice about brain injury.

The Survivor's Handbook was updated in 2006 by The Brain Trust, a nonprofit organization, now known as the Brain Injury Hope Foundation (BIHF), based in Boulder, Colorado. Donald Davis generously licensed the Survivor's Handbook to the Brain Injury Hope Foundation to publish, modify, reorganize, transform, distribute and sell. Proceeds will be used by the Brain Injury Hope Foundation to promote awareness and understanding of brain injury and to provide financial assistance to survivors of mild/moderate traumatic brain injury.

We wish to thank Elaine Gray Dumler for encouraging us to write this handbook of hope and to share our knowledge and understanding of the recovery process with our returning Warriors. Thank you to Ricardo Esparza, PhD. for his support and technical expertise especially on the post traumatic disorder definition. Thank you to Keith Schomig, lawyer and veteran, for his pro bono contribution to the section on the Rights of Veterans A special thanks goes to Tony Greco, book cover designer, to Kersti Frigell, interior illustrator, and to Dianne Nelson, interior book designer, for donating a large portion of their time and expertise to the production of this book because they believed in our vision. We also want to thank retired Army Colonel Tony Caggiano for reviewing the book from a military perspective, sharing his knowledge, and giving his stamp of approval. Thank you to Karen Carpenter, M.A., CCC-A, who provided technical assistance on the hearing section; Lisa Lanzano, MS, RD, who contributed a major portion of nutrition chapter; to Rebecca Hutchins, OD, FCOVD, who assisted with the vision chapter; and Lisa Kreber, PhD., for her expertise on physical exercise and brain injury. Thank you to Ty Miller, L.Ac., who provided the definition of acupuncturist and to Judy Haddow, M.A., CCC, for her editing and valuable input. A special thanks goes to Emerson Process Management for financial assistance for the first printing of this book.

As you can see there were many MTBI survivors and health care professionals who felt compelled to provide a better understanding of the symptoms and the recovery process of brain injury. Those who went before will be proud to know that their message of hope inspired us to write and edit this handbook of recovery especially for our returning Warriors of the current wars and all wars. It is our intention to create a greater awareness and compassion that will provide a positive environment for healing. Most importantly, to help recover the productive men and women who went to war and now need everyone's help and compassion to regain their valuable place in our society.

Dedication

This handbook of hope is dedicated to all those who are
actively serving in the current wars and to our brave
veterans and wounded Warriors from all wars, who
need the compassion and understanding of
their compatriots during recovery. Thank
you for putting your lives on the
line for Freedom
and Equality!

Mild traumatic brain injury has been labeled
the "signature injury" of the current war.[1]

CHAPTER 1

UNDERSTANDING MILD TRAUMATIC BRAIN INJURY (MTBI)

It happens in the blink of an eye. In that instant you may have experienced an injury caused by an exploding roadside bomb, a fall, a mortar blast or an automobile collision. Those who serve in combat have a greater chance of incurring a mild traumatic brain injury (MTBI) and/or post traumatic stress disorder (PTSD). Service members in the combat zone may be exposed to physical, mental, and emotional trauma on a daily basis.

Recovering from MTBI is a new assignment for those who are injured and for those caring people who want to help. The first step is to learn all you can about acquired brain injury and to accept it as a starting point—a new beginning. It is our intention to empower you with the inside knowledge and wisdom gained from those who have had MTBI and moved through the recovery process. Your own definition of "recovery" will be based on personal experience and what that means to you.

This handbook was created for you, your family, and your support system to increase awareness about brain injuries. MTBI has affected more than 300,000 military service personnel returning from the current war (April, 2009).[2] Our intention is to help you and your loved ones understand the effects of MTBI and to provide information to help you develop realistic expectations. This handbook offers suggestions on what to do to get better and resources to accelerate your healing journey. Most important, this handbook was written to inspire "hope" that you will get better; you will learn to compensate where necessary and learn new skills. When you are beyond the initial recovery stage, be open to discovering your resiliency and resourcefulness.

DEFINITION OF MTBI

A mild traumatic brain injury (MTBI) is defined as a blow or jarring of the head that results in a disruption of brain functioning. MTBI has been labeled the "signature injury" of the current war (The Associated Press, 2009). Brain injuries can range from "mild" to "severe." All brain injuries should be considered serious, and you should alert your physician about the symptoms you are having. Mild traumatic brain injuries are usually called "closed head injuries" because there is a non-penetrating injury to the brain. This type of injury can be caused by whiplash, a blast injury, or hitting the head, resulting in bruising, stretching, and shearing of the axons and/or tearing of the tissues. For the complete medical definition of MTBI, refer to **Appendix A**.

Contrary to popular belief, you DO NOT need to hit your head to sustain a mild traumatic brain injury. Although brain injuries can be caused by flying shrapnel and debris, new information indicates that concussions, due to improvised explosive devices (IEDs), may be related to blast waves. Studies being done at Johns Hopkins reveal that even if you were not hit in the head or knocked out, the indirect, powerful pressure waves caused by a bomb may affect the brain (Hagerman, 2008).[3]

MTBI OFTEN GOES UNIDENTIFIED OR MISDIAGNOSED

Brain imaging studies (MRI, CAT scan, etc.) and neurological examinations may all be normal even if you have sustained a brain injury. However, your doctor may have ordered these tests in the beginning to rule out other medical conditions. Newer imaging tests, such as, PET Scans or SPECT Scans, may be more informative for this type of injury. Many times the injury is not documented during the acute stage because the individual has physical pain that overrides the awareness of MTBI. Following a concussion or MTBI, awareness levels may be reduced and individuals may not realize that they have suffered a brain injury. Once you begin to function more normally on a physical level, the head injury becomes apparent.

The history of mild traumatic brain injury has been documented for more than a century. During the 1860's it was discovered that individuals who were injured in railway collisions suffered from brain injuries. It was believed that their symptoms were caused by "nervous shock" to the spinal cord and the brain.[4] More recent research notes that the symptoms of mild brain injury are much more serious than previously believed or shown through testing.[5]

Approximately 1.4 million people sustain a brain injury in the United States each year, and 800,000 of those are believed to be "mild traumatic brain injuries." More recent studies of individuals returning from combat in Iraq and Afghanistan reveal that at least 59% of those who were exposed to a blast were diagnosed with TBI (trau-

matic brain injury): 56% of those
moderate or severe; and 44% were
cause of Kevlar® body armor and helmets, .
uals are able to survive blast injuries—but this may
prevent MTBI. Brain injuries are cumulative in nature. In
other words, if you suffer more than one brain injury over
time, the effects may accumulate and even with a small
impact, may manifest as a more serious injury.

Although the injury may be INVISIBLE to the outside ob-
server, MTBI usually has a group of symptoms, such as
nausea, dizziness, vomiting, sleep disturbance, blurred vision, sensitivity to light and sound, fatigue, word-finding
difficulties, problems with memory, short attention span,
lowered awareness levels, decreased cognitive stamina,
etc. Emotionally, you may feel anxious, depressed, and ir-
ritable. You may lose your temper more readily and feel a
shaken sense of self—not feeling like the person you were
before. Very often there is an overlap of symptoms of acquired brain injury and post traumatic stress disorder.

DEFINITION OF POST TRAUMATIC
STRESS DISORDER (PTSD)

Survivors of TBI are particularly susceptible to major depression, generalized anxiety disorder, and post-traumatic

stress disorder. (Russoniello, et. al. 2009).[7] PTSD frequently co-exists with mild traumatic brain injury and has many of the same symptoms. PTSD is defined as a disorder that develops after a distressing psychological event that is outside typical human experience. It is characterized by re-experiencing or reliving, over and over again, painful or stressful situations. Examples of traumatic events that can cause PTSD include wars, natural disasters (hurricanes, earthquakes), accidents, physical and mental abuse.

The symptoms of PTSD may include nightmares, flashbacks, avoiding stimuli associated with the trauma, recurring memories, poor concentration, trouble sleeping, anger, exaggerated responses, and hypervigilance, among others. It is difficult to compare the symptoms of combat stress from past wars to the current time, because the effects of PTSD are often invisible. Symptoms were previously "written off" as "combat fatigue" or "shell shock" in veterans from prior wars. Now, doctors and therapists are much more aware of the psychological effects of combat and more individuals are being referred for treatment.

Since the symptoms of PTSD and MTBI can be very similar and may overlap, it is critical to identify all of your symptoms and receive all appropriate treatments. An important strategy is to undergo a neuropsychological evaluation to help differentiate between the symptoms of PTSD and MTBI. Once diagnosed, treatments may include medication, psychological counseling, eye movement desensitization and reprocessing (EMDR), somatic experiencing, brain spotting, cognitive rehabilitation, physical therapy, etc.

PTSD is a particular type of response to trauma. In the book, *Tears of a Warrior: A Family's Story of Combat and Living with* PTSD, the authors, Janet J. Seahorn, PhD, and E. Anthony Seahorn, MBA, provide excellent resources and strategies for living with PTSD. Step forward and get help to address these powerful feelings early, because there are new therapies and treatments that help to heal and control post traumatic stress disorder.

There is nothing mild about a mild traumatic brain injury!

CHAPTER 2

SIGNS AND SYMPTOMS
OF MTBI

There is nothing mild about mild traumatic brain injury! Brain injuries cause a constellation or group of symptoms that affect overall functioning. Heightened sensitivity to the environment is a common symptom of MTBI. If you have perforated your eardrums due to a blast injury, however, you may not hear as well and may have a decrease in sensitivity to sound.

The following list of symptoms are often associated with MTBI:

Physical symptoms may include:

- Headaches

- Loss of balance

- Vision problems

- Dizziness

- Loss of sex drive

- Loss of energy

- Easily fatigued

- Sensitivity to light, sound, touch

- Sleep disturbance

Emotional symptoms may include:

- Depression

- Mood swings, outbursts

- Fearfulness

- Apathy

- Low motivation

- Gullibility

- Feeling easily overloaded

- Anxiety, frustration

- Difficulty managing emotions

- Hypervigilance, exaggerated startle response

- Sense of helplessness

- Loss of sense of self, low self-esteem

- Nightmares

- Anger

Cognitive or thinking symptoms may include:

- Memory loss

- Short attention span

- Slowed thinking

- Disorientation

- Brain fatigue

- Forgetfulness

- Difficulty driving

- Word finding and spelling difficulty

- Impaired comprehension

- Inability to organize thoughts

- nability to multitask

- Inability to start or finish tasks

- Inability to inhibit certain behaviors (i.e., excessive shopping, gambling)

- Difficulty with abstract thinking

For a more detailed self-assessment, please refer to the Symptom Questionnaire for MTBI in **Appendix B**. This Questionnaire is a very valid and reliable tool used to discriminate between mild to moderate TBI and non-injured individuals. It is extremely valuable in measuring your progress over time.

It is interesting to note that both MTBI and non-injured individuals reported their greatest problems occurred in the Attention/Concentration area with the MTBI reporting the symptoms in the "Sometimes" category, whereas the non-injured marked it "Occasionally." Another interesting observation was that the second area of greatest difficulty for MTBI was in Emotional Functioning; however the second greatest difficulty for the non-injured group was Memory.

No matter where you are in your recovery, if you are experiencing any of the above symptoms, pay attention to the frequency and the intensity of a symptom. How often does it occur? Apply the frequency scale of Never, Sometimes, Frequently, or Almost Always to any symptom or behavior. For example, do you find yourself missing an appointment, getting confused, or losing your car keys more often than usual? How about tripping and falling, or forgetting driving rules more often than usual?

In addition to frequency, it is valuable to be aware of the intensity of a symptom or a behavior. For example, the sound of a person's voice may be too loud or irritating. Very often, the background noise in a restaurant can be overwhelming and uncomfortable.

EFFECTS OF BAROMETRIC PRESSURE AND ALTITUDE

You may also notice that weather patterns or elevation changes may intensify your headaches, pain and other physical symptoms. Some people will take a vacation at sea level, in order to take a "vacation" from their headaches. The correlation between high altitude and headaches has been well documented. (Serrano-Duenas, 2005: Queiroz, et. al. 2007).[1]

When changes in barometric pressure occur, individuals with MTBI complain of headaches intensifying, especially when storms move in and the barometer drops. Some countries are on the cutting edge of weather-based health forecasts that alert people to barometric pressure

_____

...ample, Canada has on-line services that forecast barometric changes. For more information go to their website www.ec.gc.ca/Envirozine.[2]

Once you are aware of the frequency and intensity of your symptoms, you can alter the environment you are in and/or your behaviors to help manage your recovery.

Remember that some symptoms can be increased by medications. You may also have side effects resulting from medications. If you have questions, do not hesitate to discuss them with your doctor.

YOU DON'T KNOW
WHAT YOU DON'T KNOW

When the brain is injured, it has to protect itself by shutting out stimuli from the outside world. In other words, it SHUTS DOWN. This may happen many times in an hour or in a day. Sometimes individuals don't recognize the symptoms of acquired brain injury, but when they start to recover from their physical injuries, they often say, "I was so injured that I wasn't aware of what I was doing or saying." At such times, your awareness levels may be low. It is difficult to know what you are missing until the brain starts to heal and the "cloud lifts."

Before an injury, many skills come automatically. It's a given; you may not have to give full attention to certain activities, for example, driving a car, riding a bike or a motorcycle, cooking, reading a book, working on the computer, following written directions or even going to familiar places. After a brain injury the "automatic pilot" may be functioning efficiently, but your speed of processing may be slower. Although you know how to do a task; you might be surprised to find out that the body is willing but the brain is slower to respond. Don't be embarrassed or fearful. Rely on people whom you trust as you move through the early healing phases of the injury.

Just imagine what it would be like
with no filter on your brain.
All the sounds, smells, images, feelings
would come crashing in at the same time.

CHAPTER 3

THE IMPORTANT ROLE
OF BRAIN FILTERS

Much of the brain's energy is used to filter out irrelevant or unnecessary information. Just imagine what it would be like with no filter on your brain. All the sounds, smells, images, and feelings would come crashing in at the same time. The overstimulation would probably paralyze you and prevent you from taking any action.

After sustaining MTBI, most of the brain's energy is diverted to basic functioning, and little is left over for filtering or censoring. Trivial or insignificant thoughts may often have the same weight in your mind as important ones. This can make decisions difficult. You may find that your brain gets stuck on an idea or phrase that keeps replaying, and this uses a great deal of brain energy.

New sensitivities can be very challenging and baffling for the injured person and their loved ones. Going into a restaurant or store where there are fluorescent lights, background music, or a great deal of visual stimuli may cause the brain to shut down. Most people say that they want to get into a quiet place and rest their brain after that experience. That is why it is so important to plan your social activities when fewer people are around and when there is less commotion.

HEARING PROBLEMS AND HYPERSENSITIVITY TO SOUND

As mentioned above, a common symptom of traumatic brain injury is hypersensitivity to sound. This is called hyperacusis. The auditory system becomes very sensitive to environmental noise, and you may discover that you have great difficulty going to restaurants, the grocery store, or social gatherings.

Many individuals report staying at home to avoid the assault and feelings of being overwhelmed in these noisy situations, or they may go out only at times when places are less crowded and less noisy. Any noise can assault and overwhelm a person with MTBI, including a vibrating refrigerator, heating system, or humming fan, etc.

An excellent accommodation for hyperacusis is ear filters. The actual name is ER 15/25 noise-dampening ear filters. These are custom-fitted earplugs, originally made for musicians, but they now have been adapted for individuals with traumatic brain injuries. Consult an audiologist at a speech and hearing clinic to obtain filters. Current studies show that filters can reduce overstimulation to the auditory system and allow you to participate in social situations without becoming overwhelmed. An advantage of using ear filters is that you can put them in for brief periods of time and take them out when you don't need them. They can be made with clear materials and are therefore less visible. The ear molds for these filters are made by an audiologist, or a specialist trained in testing hearing and treating hearing problems.

The ear is susceptible to blast injuries. Unique patterns of injury occur with bombs and explosions that are seldom seen outside of combat. The eardrum or tympanic membrane may be perforated in the blast and should be evaluated with an otologic evaluation and audiometry (hearing evaluation) to determine whether there is an injury to the ear.

Eardrums can be replaced, but observational studies over the years have shown a high rate of spontaneous healing of ruptured eardrums following blast injuries. Whether a perforated eardrum heals spontaneously depends on the size and placement of the perforation.

Two types of hearing loss are associated with blast-induced injuries. One type is called conductive hearing loss, and the second type is sensorineural hearing loss. The high-frequency sounds are more likely to be affected in blast injuries. Many individuals complain of tinnitus or ringing in the ears, and it is common to have balance problems, dizziness and/or vertigo associated with perforated eardrums. It is very important to keep the ear canal dry until the eardrum has healed.

VISION PROBLEMS AND SENSITIVITY TO LIGHT

You may notice that your eyes don't seem to be working in the same way that they did before your brain injury. Some eye doctors specialize in vision problems resulting from an acquired brain injury. They can help diagnose visual problems related to the injury and provide exercises or special glasses to help with recovery.

Because the visual changes are sometimes subtle, you may pass them off as being related to fatigue or brain fog. Aiming and focusing the eyes are linked, and that is why objects may appear to move, be seen as double, or blur in and out. Some individuals also complain that it is difficult to focus quickly from near to far or far to near.

Vision problems and cognitive deficits may compound one another. The most common complaints related to visual problems associated with brain injuries include light sensitivity, headaches, double vision, fatigue, dizziness, difficulty reading, or loss of peripheral visual fields. You may feel a heightened sensitivity to light and may even need to wear your sunglasses inside. You may have to request that fluorescent lights be turned off. Computer and reading tasks may take longer than usual, and tend to be more confusing and tiring.

A behavioral optometrist or a doctor who belongs to the Neuro-Optometric Rehabilitation Association can perform a comprehensive vision evaluation and help you determine the best course of action. Some individuals with visual deficits can benefit from specific lenses or prisms in their glasses and/or from vision therapy.

If you have vision problems associated with MTBI, this may deplete your energy and decrease your ability to perform daily living tasks. It is unrealistic to return to work until vision problems are addressed. If your job requires a great deal of reading or moving your eyes between the desk and a computer screen, you may find that your errors increase because of difficulty tracking. It is very important to address visual problems, as they can increase the recovery time.

DIZZINESS AND VERTIGO

Feelings of dizziness and nausea are common after a head injury. You may notice that these symptoms come and go depending on the activity you are doing. Dizziness may refer to distinct symptoms, one of them being vertigo. This is when you feel as though you are spinning, and sometimes you feel nauseated or like you may lose your balance. Researchers have discovered various causes for this symptom, such as problems with your inner ear, impairments in eye movements, clenching and grinding your teeth, tightness in the neck muscles, etc.

Dizziness may also originate from cervical neck injuries. The primary symptoms with this type of dizziness include feeling off balance, lightheadedness, and the sensation of floating. If you have what is called benign paroxysmal positional vertigo (BPPV), you may notice that you have a sudden attack of spinning when you turn over in bed, change your head position quickly, or reach for an item above your head. This usually lasts for less than a minute, but you may be left with feelings of nausea and dizziness for a longer time.

The Mayo Clinic developed a technique called canalith repositioning (1994). where the head is maneuvered in various positions to help eliminate the dizziness. This is accomplished by moving the calcium crystals in the inner ear.[1] Medications that can help dizziness are also available. Be sure to consult with your doctor to see if you need a referral to an ear doctor who specializes in traumatic dizziness and/or an eye doctor who specializes in traumatic vision syndrome.

CHANGES IN ENERGY RESERVE AFTER INJURY

Healing takes a tremendous amount of energy. The diagram in *Figure* 1 illustrates functioning before and after the injury. It shows how the uninjured brain can perform many activities that are physical, cognitive, and emotional throughout the day, and still have a reserve of energy. After a brain injury, it takes more energy to deal with cognitive and emotional issues, leaving little or no reserve.

The brain uses more energy than any other organ in the body. Before you were injured, you had a pool of reserve energy available when you overextended yourself. Following your injury, nearly all of your energy is required to perform the most basic functions just to get through the day. If you are continuing to work, you may find that when you get home, you must rest and not engage in other activities as before.

THE ENERGY PIE

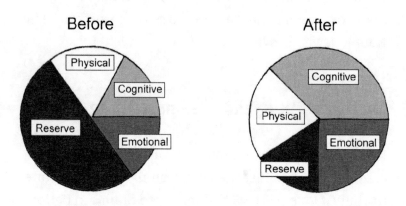

Figure 1
© Mary Lou Acimovic, MA, CCC-Sp

Your energy reserves at this point are almost nonexistent. When you push too much you may reach overload,

and the extreme fatigue may cause your bra
to shut down. This exhaustion can also amplify ... of your
symptoms, and cause an emotional reaction.

Almost Immediately after an injury it becomes clear that
you don't have the same amount of energy that you previously did. It is important to emphasize the need for rest
and conserving energy. For a while you may be unable to
do as much as you used to and may need to take time out
for rest—Brain Rest. Lay down during the day for naps.
Even if you don't sleep, resting your head and lying down
may make a significant difference in your recovery.

Most likely, your brain may be processing more slowly, and the mechanisms that you could previously depend on as your "automatic pilot" may be temporarily damaged or not there to protect you as they did before.

CHAPTER 4

BABY, YOU CAN
DRIVE MY CAR

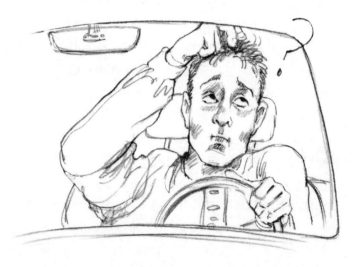

Regardless of whether your injury was caused by a blast, a motor vehicle accident or sports-related activity, it may take time before you feel comfortable behind the wheel.

iduals report that it is more difficult to
. This is typical. The speed of traffic, the confusing activity in your peripheral vision, and the hypervigilant effort necessary for driving can overwhelm you. Being so overwhelmed can cause stress, increase headaches, and affect your reaction time.

It is important to note again, "You don't know what you don't know"—meaning that you may think you are still capable of driving but discover that you should postpone driving for a while. For example, when you come to a four-way stop sign, you may forget what to do. Or, you might notice that, when your eyes leave the road and you glance from left to right, you may get distracted longer than usual. Please pay attention to your level of awareness. Take a family member or a friend for a ride for a second opinion.

Most likely, your brain may be processing more slowly, and the mechanisms that you could previously depend on as your "automatic pilot" may be temporarily damaged or not there to protect you as they did before. It may be unsafe to do two things at the same time, such as driving while looking at the scenery, talking on a cell phone or to a passenger. This is a perfect example of multitasking skills that were previously taken for granted, but may now be compromised.

Your brain may struggle to register all the necessary information that driving requires. This previously occurred at lightning speed without much conscious thought. Now, processing may occur in a slow fashion. Don't be surprised if you find yourself lost while driving in an area you've known for years. Avoid driving when you are tired!

Many individuals carry their cell phones with them while driving in case they have to PULL OVER to call someone to help orient them to their location or give them directions. You may also benefit from a GPS locator system that gives verbal directions.

Here are some options to help with the transition back to driving:

- Arrange to ride with a friend.

- Ask a friend to drive you in your car.

- Check out the bus routes.

- Use taxicabs or special transit.

- Use roads that are less crowded, and don't drive during rush hour. It may take longer, but you will feel safer.

- Map out your route in advance, even if you have driven this route many times. It will be one less step for your brain to worry about.

- Explore the possibility of carpooling to your care providers with other patients. If you can coordinate appointments with another person, you can alternate driving and have company on the ride.

- Explore facilities in your area that specialize in teaching driving strategies to individuals who are returning to the road after an accident or physical injury. They can check out your reaction time.

My Thoughts and Observations

Appearances can be deceiving. You are dealing with
a different person even though they may look the same.
Be compassionate, supportive, and patient.

CHAPTER 5

HELPFUL TIPS FOR FAMILY, FRIENDS, AND LOVED ONES

This will be a time of challenge for you, too. The person you know and love has changed. These changes may be drastic, or they may be subtle. It may take time for the full effect of the injury to set in. When it does, this person will need all of the unconditional love and support you can offer. Your acceptance will greatly support their recovery.

You may feel anger, frustration, impatience, and confusion. Try your best to understand and accept what has happened. Accompanying the person to their health appointments and listening to what the health care providers have to say will often help you to better understand the nature of the injury.

to what the injured person is saying, and p— their behavior. Remember that their communication skills may have been impaired. A person with MTBI may not be able to tell you what is wrong. Recognize that their brain does not work like it did before the injury and because of this, they may have trouble expressing what is needed right now. Lower your expectations of their ability and energy level.

Avoid telling the injured person that they "look fine." Appearances can be deceiving, and although they may look fine, they don't feel that way. Remember that you're dealing with a different person now. Be prepared for emotional swings, low energy, absentmindedness, and a constant struggle to maintain balance. Be compassionate, supportive, and patient.

One key symptom of MTBI is the inability to initiate actions. For example, you may know what you want to do, know the steps to complete the task, but find that you are unable to physically begin. This is known as a **lack of initiation**. It is very confusing and people often times mistake it for laziness. If you and your family member understand the nature of this symptom, there are rehab techniques to breakthrough this inability to get started.

You may also find that your family member spends money impulsively, but does not realize it and has a lack of insight regarding the overall financial impact. Be sure to monitor your loved one's spending habits and participate in balancing the checkbook to avioid overdrawing accounts.

You will probably have to do more for them than ever before. Even simple tasks will seem too much for them some days. Helping with errands and household chores, dealing with insurance companies, and offering a supportive hug can all make a world of difference. Don't set any limits on their recovery. Throw out the old schedule, forget old expectations, and embrace the person exactly the way they are right now.

It may take a while to learn how to avoid feeling overloaded. Be patient and help them, but don't force them. They may have good days, followed by days when they are unable to function as well. This is normal, so try to be understanding and supportive.

As much as you may want to, you cannot "fix" the brain injury. Give them the space they need to heal and encourage them to talk with others who understand.

You will find that it is helpful to speak with others in your situation or to consult with a counselor for your own needs. Do take care of yourself so that you can be supportive to the injured person. Remember to take personal time to recharge and renew that wonderful, caring gift that you have to offer. Ask friends and family to share daily activities, such as driving to appointments. Learn to pace yourself and ask yourself what you need throughout the day.

This is part of your own recovery path as well. Allow yourself to accept help from others. As you provide a safe place for them to heal, look for the gifts that everyone will receive. Focus on the little successes along the way, because with a hopeful heart, you will see positive outcomes that you never expected.

My Thoughts and Observations

It takes the strength and courage of a true warrior
to recover from a brain injury that has shaken
your entire being.

CHAPTER 6

NEW ATTITUDES
AND LATITUDES

One of the most frustrating aspects of having MTBI is that there is no apparent wound or readily visible sign of your injury. People will tell you how good you look, how you don't seem injured, or encourage you to believe that you are healed before you are. Please understand that they mean well.

There may even be times when you doubt the extent of your injury and try to continue your life as you did in the past, only to find that you can't function the way you did previously. This is a typical realization. Now is the time to be patient with yourself. Your new full-time job is healing your brain injury. Following are some guidelines to make your recovery easier and quicker.

BALANCE AND STRUCTURE

Take time to grieve your loss—the loss of who you were before the injury. We have been there, and we know how devastating this feels. Everything seems changed, including the way people relate to you.

Don't try to ignore it. Go ahead and feel the hurt and anger. Discuss your feelings with a friend, family member, therapist or counselor who can help you process the effects of the injury.

Create a new structure for your life. Plan your days and activities carefully. Set up a routine that works for you. Try not to overload yourself by scheduling too many things on any one day. Remember, activities that were easily accomplished before now require a great deal of planning and effort. Try to give yourself at least two or three "lighter load days" during the week.

Block out time for rest and sleep. Pay careful attention to your diet, and be sure to eat healthy foods and drink plenty of water. Eat before you get hungry. Don't go for long periods without eating—the brain needs energy to heal and function. You can't drive a car without gas. The same goes for our bodies and especially the control center—the brain.

It has been noted that weight gain is common following brain injury. Keep yourself on a healthy eating and sleeping schedule and understand your body's needs. Your body gives you clues and signals all the time, such as when you are about to reach your maximum threshold. Be sure to listen and take good care of yourself.

AVOID OVERLOAD AND BURNOUT

Make a list of things that cause you to feel overloaded, and devise a way to avoid them or get more control over them. Your therapist will have experience with this and can help you develop a plan.

During our busy life schedules, we are used to multitasking. Prior to your injury, you may have been able to do many things at the same time. However, you may now find it necessary to create a list and prioritize tasks in order of importance. A common symptom includes being overwhelmed with activities of daily life. That is why it is so important to pace yourself throughout the day, limit the activities that you are doing, and focus on the most important things you want to complete.

There will be people who do not understand what you are going through and who perhaps may even deny that you have been injured. Situations involving these types of people can be especially frustrating. Try to avoid these situations, if possible. Do your best to minimize the presence of difficult people in your life. Healing takes a lot of energy. (Is there a pattern here?) Slow everything in your life down until you find a pace that's comfortable for you.

Everyone recovers from injuries at his or her own pace. Your experience will be unique, and when you have bad days, remember that better ones will follow them. Setbacks are a natural part of the recovery process.

STAIR-STEP RECOVERY MODEL

The recovery from mild traumatic brain injury can take quite some time. Although many individuals recover within the first 90 days, the initial healing time is typically 18-24 months. Many say that they still notice recovery between 3 to 5 years post-injury. The first 90 days is called the period of "rapid spontaneous recovery," when the brain is going through spontaneous healing. Brain injuries recover in what is known as a stair-step recovery which is illustrated in *Figure* 2 on the next page.

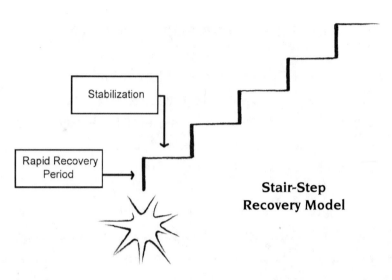

Figure 2

Recovery moves through a series of steps where you will most likely notice a rapid recovery period followed by a stabilization period. This pattern repeats itself over time. When you are in the stabilization, or "flat" part of the stair step, you may think that you will stay as you are and not continue to recover. The majority of individuals find, however, that they continue to see improvements across many areas of cognitive functioning over many years. This is a positive aspect of the recovery process. By understanding the stair-step recovery model, it gives you the realistic hope you need over time to stay with the healing process.

SLEEP, REST, AND SLEEP SOME MORE

Oh, yes, sleep. Never before has sleep been so important. Now rest and sleep are essential for your body and mind to function at even the most basic level. Sleep as much as you can, whenever and wherever you need to. Listen to your body, and when it says it is tired, allow it to rest.

Give yourself lots of time during the day to rest and nap, and plan on at least ten hours of sleep each night. Remember, you have little reserve energy—only a limited amount each day—and that is greatly affected by how much rest you have had.

You may experience sleep disruption as a result of the injury. Explore ways to overcome this with your healthcare

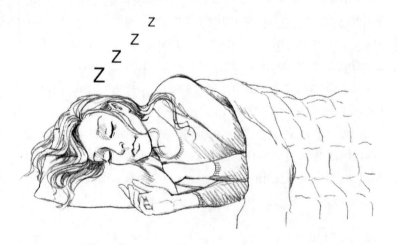

providers. This is very important, because lack of sleep will intensify your symptoms and may extend the amount of time it takes to recover.

WRITE IT DOWN

Memory and multitasking are areas frequently affected by MTBI. This can be very frustrating and even frightening. Write yourself notes about everything important. Don't try to keep things in your head the way you did before your injury. Carry an appointment book, electronic or cell phone organizer with you at all times. At home, keep a large, plain calendar in clear view in the kitchen. Refer to it frequently to remind you about appointments. Transfer appointments from your appointment book to the calendar in large, clearly printed letters. Ask for help from family or friends if keeping your calendar is too difficult. Sometimes people feel disoriented to the time of day, and they use a beeping reminder watch or set their cell phone to alert them a half hour before an appointment.

Maybe you used to keep lots of things juggled in your head. Maybe you have never missed an appointment. You may find that this happens now—or you may, for example, show up at the right time on the wrong day. Don't force your brain to remember things that you can write down. Ask your doctors and therapists to write down directions and other information for you.

You may also find that you don't remember things that you have said or done. Don't panic! Ask others to be patient with you, and remember to be patient with yourself. You will improve over time. Don't get caught up in the frustration of the moment.

It is helpful to keep a record or a health journal of your medical progress and the treatments that are helping. It also will help you document your reaction to different medications and treatments. Refer to the medication record in **Appendix C**.

My Thoughts and Observations

Your recovery will put you in touch with yourself
in a whole new way. Very often, this type
of injury gives you time to reflect
on your life and on what is most important.

CHAPTER 7

HEALING IS A
FULL-TIME JOB

Although it may not be visible, you have sustained a powerful, life-changing injury. Don't try to make yourself well, based on your own timetable. Healing the brain is a slow process, and you can extend your recovery time by trying to do too much, too soon.

If you have been injured while on duty, a profile will be completed that will outline the tasks that you will, and will not be expected to perform. You may be assigned to light duty before returning to the field. If you are working, it may be important to let your superior officers, supervisors and co-workers know what you're going through. It will be difficult for you to function the way you did previously and their understanding and cooperation will be essential. You may need to take a furlough, leave of absence or assume less-complicated job responsibilities. You may also need time off from work for your health appointments.

IT IS WHAT IT IS!

Accept the fact that you are injured, and treat yourself like you might treat an injured loved one—with lots of pampering and compassion. It's normal to have mood swings, to grieve the loss of your "old self," and to feel adrift. Remain flexible. It is what it is! The old concept of "no pain, no gain" does not work in healing a brain injury—your brain needs rest, and **you should not push yourself beyond your physical or cognitive limits**. You will know when the time is right to go to the next level of activity and thinking.

If you are taking good care of yourself, you are spending a lot of time resting. Meditation, biofeedback, and breathing exercises can be extremely helpful as well. Try to quiet the mind and focus on a word or object while breathing deeply. A typical breathing exercise is to breathe in to the count of four and breathe out to the count of eight. Repeat eight to ten times. Breathing exercises have been known to calm the anxious mind and lower blood pressure.

Visualization is another way to quiet your brain and help your body feel better. Use your own memory tapes to recall happy occasions. Use positive images to redirect your thinking. Music is also a powerful mood changer. The companionship of a pet has been shown to be "good medicine." Various organizations, such as, Freedom Dogs, are enlisting canines to assist troops at home and abroad. (www.petside.com).[1]

TRY IT—YOU MIGHT LIKE IT

Success stories happen every day with this type of injury. People who have never even thought of writing, have written books after their injury. Some have pursued careers in the arts, and others have explored new occupations through vocational rehabilitation. You may discover talents that you never knew you had.

Did you ever think of learning to play that musical instrument you always wanted to try or you set aside in your younger years? Many of these activities integrate both sides of the brain and promote healing in a more profound way.

HELP ME HELP MYSELF

Many of us with brain injuries were very self-sufficient prior to our injury. People came to us for help. But now that's all changed, and we are the ones who need help. Asking for help is a new behavior. We don't want to impose, appear weak, or feel obligated to others.

A natural reaction is to deny it, because we don't want anyone to know that we are not capable. Denial is hoping that it will disappear by itself. It is a self-defense mechanism. However, in the case of MTBI, if you don't move beyond this level of denial, you may miss the fast track to healing in those early months of recovery.

Your willingness to ask for help opens the door to healing. Asking for help is a sign of courage and strength. We hope that the people closest to us can read our minds, but most of the time they can't. So, tell them what you need. Allowing people to help you is a gift to them.

WHO CAN HELP?

It's important to talk with people who understand what you are going through. Doctors and therapists can be helpful and are great listeners. You may also need family or couple's counseling to help your significant others to understand your feelings about this radical change in your life. Therapy also gives them a chance to discuss their concern and confusion.

Try to find a brain injury support group in your area. Ask your therapist or health-care providers if they know of any. Contact your state Brain Injury Association, or the National Brain Injury Association at 1-800-444-6443, or at www.biausa.org, for more information. Refer to the **Resources section** in the back of the handbook for an expanded list.

Services are available to help you with the day-to-day chores that can become overwhelming. Many supermarkets offer shopping and delivery service. You can also find people to run errands and cook meals for you. Friends can help with phone calls, car pooling the kids around, and other obligations.

If you are able to use the Internet to explore brain injury Web sites or chat rooms, you may find useful information. Reach out to your community. If you are a member of a church or a spiritual group, ask those individuals for help.

Remember to delegate—simplify—dump!

Having a coordinated treatment team and plan will expedite your recovery. Make sure your providers have expertise with brain injury.

CHAPTER 8

MEDICAL PROFESSIONALS
WHO TREAT MTBI

For those with MTBI, recovery is a full-time job. The first part of that job is to find capable health care providers who understand MTBI. They will help make your recovery faster and easier. But do not expect a "quick fix." Although you can't see the extent of the injury to the brain, it is there, and it will take time to heal.

When choosing providers, be direct in asking questions such as, "Are you familiar with mild traumatic brain injury?" or, "Have you had experience treating MTBI?" and "What is your approach in treating MTBI?"

Based on their answers, you will have a better idea if this provider is right for you. Trust your instincts!

e are many kinds of therapists and doctors who can
e helpful.

Doctors include:

- Your family doctor.

- Neurologists treat the nervous system.

- Osteopaths are physicians who use a hands on approach to treat muscular-skeletal problems.

- Chiropractors manipulate joints of the body.

- Psychiatrists are physicians who can prescribe medication.

- Physiatrists are physicians who prescribe rehabilitative therapies and medications.

- Naturopathic doctors use natural methods or modalities to heal.

- Ophthalmologists and optometrists specialize in visual evaluation and treatment.

- Find physicians who specialize in MTBI.

Therapists include:

- Psychologists provide individual/marital/family counseling focused on developing coping skills, releasing trauma, and improving emotional, and social functioning.

- Physical therapists use hands-on mobilization of muscles and joints.

- Speech-Language pathologists, or occupational therapists provide cognitive rehabilitation to help retrain your brain and improve memory through specific exercises; as well as, teach you ways to compensate for deficits while you recover.

- Neuropsychologists perform extensive testing to document how your brain is functioning cognitively and psychologically.

- Massage therapists use manipulation of the soft tissue structures of the body to reduce stress and relax the body and mind.

- Cranial sacral therapists use very light touch to heal and balance the cranial sacral system in the body.

- Neurofeedback therapists use EEG biofeedback equipment to provide feedback about how your brain is functioning and help you alter these frequencies and promote healing.

- Biofeedback specialists use sensitive instruments to measure physical responses (e.g. muscular tension, temperature, breathing, fight-or-flight responses, etc.) and then provide feedback and strategies to help alter the body's response to stress.

- Acupuncturists place pins the thickness of a fine hair into specific acupuncture points that are known to assist with rejuvenating the brain, calming headaches and relieving pain.

- Vision therapists use a type of physical therapy for the eyes and brain to help the eyes work together, track better, etc.

- Pilates instructors teach a series of non-impact exercises designed by Joseph Pilates to develop strength, flexibility, balance, and inner awareness.

- Vocational counselors assist with finding a new vocation and/or retrain you for work.

- Other alternative therapy providers, such as hypnotherapists, may also be helpful.

WHERE TO START WITH TREATMENT PLANS

Because MTBI affects so many areas of functioning—seeing, hearing, physical movement, thinking ability, emotions, balance and coordination, etc., it can be confusing where to begin. Just remember, the main rule is to find someone who has experience and has treated MTBI.

One starting point is to go to your physician, a neurologist or a doctor of physical medicine also known as a physiatrist. Your doctor may refer you for further evaluation. Regardless of where you start, you will need to seek out care that is defined by the symptoms you have. It often requires a medical team who work together on your behalf.

Many individuals address the pain first by seeing an osteopathic physician or a physical therapist. Osteopathic physicians can provide cranial/sacral treatments to relieve headaches and pain. Physical therapists decrease pain, improve muscular strength and endurance.

If you have difficulties thinking, contact a speech/language pathologist or occupational therapist who specializes in the treatment of cognitive problems associated with neurological disorders. You may need to see a neuropsychologist, who can evaluate, identify, and differentiate the cognitive problems from the emotional problems. Someone who specializes in trauma release work, such as a psychologist trained in Eye Movement Desensitization and Reprocessing (EMDR), brain spot-

tic experiencing, will help release the trauma and teach coping techniques. Optometrists who specialize in post-traumatic vision syndrome can give you eye exercises.

You may benefit from medications to decrease some symptoms, such as post-concussive headaches, depression, anxiety, etc. Hyperbaric Oxygen is another treatment that individuals have found to be helpful.

This is not an inclusive list, but once you begin to see healthcare professionals who work with MTBI, they will direct you to others who will complement your treatment program. It often requires a multidisciplinary treatment program to meet all of your needs.

A word of caution. Many health-care professionals are not trained or familiar with the symptoms of MTBI. It is important to have a primary care physician (PCP) with this experience in MTBI to coordinate the types and timing of your treatments. Have your providers talk with one another so that everyone is working together. You may want to ask for a meeting between yourself and your providers. Make sure that you take your medication record and calendar with you to every therapy and doctor's appointment. A form has been provided in **Appendix D** to list the names, addresses, and telephone numbers of your healthcare providers. Be sure to keep this list updated.

A WORD ABOUT MEDICATIONS

Some of your doctors will likely prescribe medications. Keep a list of the names, dosages, and schedules of all medications you take, and be sure to give this list to each provider. You may find that you react differently to medicines since your injury. Some studies show that chemicals in the brain that are released during the traumatic process can be stabilized with appropriate medications. These medications can be beneficial in accelerating the healing process. A medication record chart is provided in **Appendix C**.

It is very important to eat healthy foods to help the brain function efficiently. Feed your brain with protein snacks throughout the day.

CHAPTER 9

FEED YOUR BODY, FEED YOUR BRAIN:

Nutritional Tips to Speed Recovery

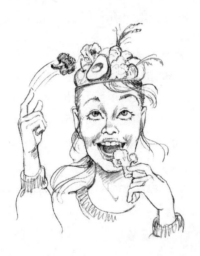

A good diet during the recovery from a brain injury is highly beneficial. Scientists know that deficiencies in certain nutrients and chemicals can cause disruptions in brain functioning and the ability to think clearly. The brain uses calories to function. When someone sustains a brain injury, it is necessary to eat enough nutritional calories to help the brain function efficiently.

NUTRITIONAL TIPS FOR HEAD INJURIES

- Eat small meals every three to four hours.

- Keep small baggies of healthy snacks with you during the day to boost your energy (nuts, trail mix, apples, cheese, hard-boiled eggs, etc.). Ask a member of your family or support group to make these for you and put them in a small cooler in your car.

- Balance small meals with a combination of protein, such as fish, lean meats, nuts and beans with healthy fats and oils from avocados, seeds, and nuts along with carbohydrates found in vegetables, fresh fruits, and grains. Avoid eating carbohydrates by themselves if you have blood sugar concerns. Many individuals report that sugar and chocolate increase headaches; therefore, eat sweets sparingly.

- Eat moderately. Do not overeat (this may make you sleepy and/or tired).

- Eat by the clock. If your brain/body signals are not working well, set a timer, watch alarm or a mobile phone to alert you that it's time to eat.

- Try to eat around the same time every day. The body does best when it is on a routine schedule.

Shopping and preparing meals take a lot of energy. The grocery store is a very difficult environment when you have a head injury because of the lights, visual stimulation, and sounds.

HELPFUL SHOPPING AND MENU IDEAS

- Create a shopping list of items you use regularly. Photocopy this list so that you can circle the items you need to purchase the next time. If you go to the same store each week, plan your list to follow the order of the aisles. (e.g. fresh foods usually line the walls or periphery of the grocery store, with packaged, canned, and frozen foods in the center aisles). This will help you conserve energy so that you won't have to make trips back and forth across the store. A magnetized notepad posted on the refrigerator is a time saver for writing down the food items to get during your next shopping trip.

- If you must go to the commissary or Post Exchange (PX), try to choose a time when it is less crowded and less noisy. In the beginning, enlist the help of neighbors or friends to pick up your shopping list when they are making a trip to the grocery store.

- If you are sensitive to noise and light, wear earplugs or filters and/or tinted glasses when shopping.

- Shop when you are well-fed. You will make smarter food choices when you are not starving as you shop and your focus and attention will be sharper.

- Develop a list of your favorite fast, easy meal ideas. Keep this posted on your fridge or inside a cupboard door for easy access.

- Keep menus simple—avoid recipes with elaborate steps or unusual ingredients that aren't familiar to you.

- When preparing meals, always make extra to store in the refrigerator for the next day or two, or freeze them. Put portions of foods into plastic or glass containers, and cover them with lids or plastic wrap.

- Throw protein foods out after three days in the refrigerator. Always practice safe food handling. Visit http://www.foodsafety.gov for further information.

- After a brain injury some people lose their sense of smell, and it is very important to be alert to the expiration dates on food.

WHAT ABOUT VITAMINS AND SUPPLEMENTS?

There are many articles on the Internet regarding the nutrition-brain connection.

Following is a list of supplements that some people have found to be helpful:

- Multivitamins

- Calcium/magnesium/vitamin D

- Omega-3 fish oil

- Probiotics (lactobacillus acidophilus plus bifidobacterium bifidus)

- Brain Vibrance (Crayhon Research Products: www.crayhonresearch.com)

- Coenzyme Q10

- Phosphatidyl serine (PS)

- Acetyl L-carnitine

- Vitamin C

- B vitamins

You should consult your physician or healthcare provider for an individualized program of supplementation. By eat-

…ou are laying a good foundation for recovery of
… body and brain.

FOODS TO AVOID

Try to avoid eating the following foods:

- Alcohol

- Caffeine

- Salty foods

- Excessive sweets and candy

Warning:

You may find that if you drink alcohol following your injury, it may have a stronger effect than before because
your tolerance level has changed. Alcohol may interact
with prescription medications. Some people may turn to
alcohol or other addictive substances to medicate themselves for physical or emotional pain. It has been said
that there should be no bottom line here. The use of
these drugs in an already disrupted physiological system
will further induce neurological and cognitive decline.
They should be avoided by survivors of TBI." (Jay, 2000).[1]

My Thoughts and Observations

A little brain exercise daily goes a long way
toward recovery. Think of it this way, cognitive
exercise stimulates brain functioning
just as aerobic exercise builds body fitness.

CHAPTER 10

HOW TO IMPROVE MEMORY
AND THINKING SKILLS

WHO CAN TEST AND TREAT
BRAIN FUNCTIONS?

Cognitive therapists and/or neuropsychologists can test your brain functioning to assess the areas of strength and weakness. Neuropsychological testing is highly advanced and evaluates both the emotional and cognitive factors related to brain injury. Cognitive therapists, who treat brain injuries, are usually speech/language pathologists or occupational therapists. They can provide exercises to help strengthen brain functions, such as attention and concentration, memory, logical reasoning, problem solving, speed of processing, initiating activities, reading, math skills, etc. Some of the exercises use pencil and paper and some use software on the computer. Search the Internet for brain fitness websites to improve memory and cognitive skills. Refer to the Resources section in the back of the book.

You can purchase books that contain cognitive exercises at your local book store. The Resources section in the back of the book contains a list of recommended books on improving brain function. It is good to exercise your brain, however, it is important not to do these for long periods of time in the beginning, as this may overload your brain and cause an increase in your symptoms. Many times throughout this book, you will notice that we recommend a timer. It is an excellent way to remind you when to take a break. Start with a maximum of five to ten minutes of brain exercises, until you know your brain's tolerance. If you start to get a headache or you have the sensation that your brain feels full, stop the task and consider putting an ice pack on the back of your neck. Also, if there are brain-related activities that you find difficult in the beginning, your cognitive therapist can suggest ways for you to compensate until your brain is ready to advance.

BRAIN STRETCHERS

When you are able to think without tiring, the following activities can help the brain form new information pathways and perform more efficiently. Your providers may have additional suggestions.

Crossword puzzles give your word-finding skills a workout. Frequently, word retrieval skills are affected by the injury, and remembering even simple words can be tough. You will quickly graduate to more challenging levels. Take breaks and consider finishing a difficult crossword puzzle the next day. You will be surprised how quickly the answers show up after you have rested or have had a good night's sleep. Cognitive Therapists can provide specific rehabilitation programs to improve brain functioning. You may find a list of Cognitive Therapists on www.asha.org.

A little brain exercise daily goes a long way toward recovery. Think of it this way, cognitive exercise stimulates brain functioning just as aerobic exercise builds body fitness. Watching Wheel of Fortune on TV can be an entertaining way of exercising your recall skills. There are programs available on the Internet designed to improve cognition, speed of processing, and memory skills. For example, www.puzzlersparadise.com, www.CogniFit.com, www.braingle.com and www.Lumosity.com. Many people also find the Nintendo DS Lite with Brain Age software to be convenient and portable.

Sudoku puzzles are an excellent way to work on sequencing, planning, and problem solving. These are great exercises because you can stop and pick them up later without losing your place. Start with the easy level and build up to the more challenging levels.

Logic puzzles help break down the thinking process into steps. The rapid speed at which your brain used to come to conclusions may have been affected, and trying to make those "snap" decisions now can be difficult. Logic puzzles use reasoning and brain focus to draw conclusions.

Card games and board games provide social opportunities for laughter and companionship. Some games to consider include Scrabble, Scattergories, Taboo, and Rushhour. Card games such as Crazy Eights, Gin Rummy, and Bridge are excellent for sharpening the brain. Also consider Solitaire; use playing cards rather than the computer, as it exercises your logic and eye-hand coordination. The card game called Speed improves many of the skills mentioned above.

WHAT DOES EXERCISE HAVE TO DO WITH IT?

Physical exercise is an important part of recovery from a brain injury, even if it's walking a short distance a few times a week. Be sure to consult your doctor and/or physical therapist before returning to physical exercise. In the early stages of recovery, be cautious when engaging in physical activities where the brain may be jarred (e.g., running, horseback riding, skiing, mountain biking and motocross). It is also important to assess whether you can process information and react as quickly as you could previously. In activities that require rapid reaction times, it may be difficult to meet the physical challenges until your reaction time improves.

We all know that physical exercise makes us feel better because it alleviates stress and increases the flow of endorphins. Dr. Ratey, author of *Spark: The Revolutionary New Science of Exercise and and the Brain*, states that physical exercise can sharpen your thinking, improve memory skills, and prepare the brain for learning. He also talks about the many scientifically proven benefits of aerobic exercise and emphasizes the relationship of exercise and mood elevation.[1]

Current research on exercise and brain functioning reveals the following:

- Aerobic exercise increases blood flow to the brain.

- Exercise increases the level of brain-derived neurotropic factor (BDNF), which is like brain fertilizer and can help with integrity of neurons and other neuronal structures.

- Exercise enhances mood, most likely due to the release of endorphins.

My Thoughts and Observations

Biofeedback has been shown to improve
anxiety responses and may allow you to go into
a relaxation response rather than a stress response.

CHAPTER 11

WHAT IS BIOFEEDBACK
AND NEUROFEEDBACK?

Biofeedback and EEG neurofeedback are important treatment techniques that are being used in the VA system to assist recovering veterans. Biofeedback/neurofeedback was studied by Dr. Eugene Peniston (1991, 1993) for the treatment of combat-related, post traumatic stress disorder and substance abuse.[1] These modalities have also been identified as being successful in the treatment of MTBI (Ayers,1987; Bounias and Laibow, 2001; Thornton, 2000).[2]

Currently, there are numerous biofeedback and neurofeedback training programs for optimal performance that have shown good preliminary results in reducing or eliminating symptoms of TBI and PTSD (Russiniello, 2009).[3] Proactive methods to help troops develop a resiliency to combat stress are being implemented and studied by Pyne and Gevirtz (2009).[4]

Biofeedback is the use of sensitive instruments to measure physical responses in the body and feed them back to you in order to help alter your body's responses. You can observe the feedback on a computer screen or listen to sound feedback.

BIOFEEDBACK TREATMENT OPTIONS

Different types of biofeedback are used to treat various physical and emotional problems. For example:

- Electromyographic (EMG) biofeedback may be used to treat muscular tension headaches as well as neck pain, jaw pain, etc.

- Temperature biofeedback helps you learn to increase blood flow into various parts of the body. Having a head injury may cause temperature dysregulation. Many individuals report feeling very hot or very cold.

- Electrodermal response (EDR) is a way to measure the body's tendency to go into a fight-or-flight response. This may happen after a traumatic event, such as a blast or car accident.

- Pneumographic biofeedback (breathing biofeedback) is a modality used to measure chest versus abdominal breathing. This can help you learn to breathe more deeply and regularly to improve your relaxation response.

- Heart rate variability biofeedback entrains the cardiovascular and physiological systems which may positively affect conditions, such as, depression and anxiety.

- EEG neurofeedback or brain-wave biofeedback is a form of biofeedback in which surface electrodes are placed on the scalp to measure specific brain-wave frequencies and provide feedback to the individual. You may learn to suppress or enhance specific brain-wave frequencies, thus enabling you to learn to focus, relax, and increase flexibility of thinking.

- The primary brain-wave frequencies that are measured include delta, theta, alpha, low beta, and beta. Different brain-wave frequencies are associated with various states and various disorders. For example, individuals with traumatic brain injuries frequently have an abundance of theta waves, or low-frequency brain waves. Attention deficit disorders also reveal high levels of theta. The goal of this treatment is to teach individuals to move flexibly in and out of certain brain-wave states in order to enhance performance. If theta levels are too high and you cannot focus, you may want to learn to suppress that wave and increase alpha and beta, which will allow you to be more focused and present. Many of the neurofeedback protocols used with TBI and PTSD also involve sensorimotor rhythm (SMR) training.

TREATMENT TECHNIQUES

In conjunction with visual and auditory feedback from the biofeedback equipment and brain-wave machines, individuals are encouraged to practice daily techniques to enhance their skill levels.

Following are some of the most successful techniques:

- Progressive muscle relaxation

- Deep muscle relaxation

- Breathing and muscle awareness

- Autogenic relaxation

- Visual imagery

- Open-focus training

- Systematic desensitization

- Short relaxation forms (e.g., quieting response, body stress scanning)

- Carryover techniques to bring the strategies into everyday living situations

BENEFITS GAINED FROM BIOFEEDBACK AND NEUROFEEDBACK

The benefits of biofeedback depend on the skills you want to learn. For example, you may learn to warm your hands, which may, in turn, lower your blood pressure or decrease migraine headaches. By learning to relax the muscles in your face, neck, shoulders, and back, you may be able to eliminate or decrease tension headaches, jaw pain, back pain, or clenching and grinding of your teeth. By learning to go into a relaxation response rather than a stress response, you may decrease anxiety. The benefits of neurofeedback are many; for example, you may learn to alter your brain-wave frequencies to decrease foggy thinking and increase clarity and cognitive stamina. It is important to see a provider who is certified by the Biofeedback Certification Institute of America (www.bcia.org).

Give yourself all the time you need to heal.
Avoid putting yourself on a timetable.
Your recovery is a major life transformation.

CHAPTER 12

HOW LONG BEFORE
I'M BETTER?

Where is the magic wand when we need it? Recovery time varies from person to person, although it is never as fast as we would like it to be. One rule of thumb is that about 75% of people with MTBI will improve substantially within the first 3 to 6 months. However, the recovery from mild traumatic brain injury can take quite some time. Typically the initial healing time is 18-24 months. Many say that they still notice recovery between 3 to 5 years post-injury. But, don't be surprised or discouraged if your symptoms linger. You will get better over time especially with cognitive therapy and exercises.

THE PROCESS OF RECOVERY

To some, the word "recovery" means getting better, regaining what you lost, the pain goes away and the brain

is as sharp and attentive as it was before the accident. However, every brain injury is as varied as the recovery process because of the uniqueness of who you are. A brain injury is unlike all other injuries.

In the morning, you may be able to do two or three things at one time and by afternoon, you can barely focus on one thing and follow it through without being distracted. Or, you start out in the morning and tasks become more difficult as the day goes on. There are many things that you can do to adjust to the new demands. One of the most beneficial things is to sleep at least 8 hours a night. In the early stages of recovery, sleep may be what your body and brain need most of all. Give in to it because that is a natural healing response. Perhaps your body rhythm is off and you have difficulty sleeping at night. Consider taking naps throughout the day whenever you feel tired. Eventually, your body will adjust to normal sleep and awake patterns.

When injured, the brain shuts down to protect itself. As the recovery process continues, the brain wakes up and the fog lifts. If you haven't started the rehabilitation process, it is now time for the gentle help of cognitive, physical and emotional rehabilitation. There are many articles and books about people who have made miracu-

lous recoveries from head injuries and gone on to thrive and live happy and productive lives. In fact, some individuals actually report that they are better than they were prior to the injury because they now understand how the brain works. They have learned how to stimulate brain functioning, how to exercise their bodies efficiently, how to judge the amount of sleep they need, and how to feed their bodies nutritionally to help them maintain healthy lifestyles.

Consider this. We are always growing and changing. The cells of the body are constantly being replaced according to their own schedule and demand. As we mature, we may change our beliefs, attitudes and life strategies which are influenced by experiences, relationships, and current situations. We may change our preferences for foods, music, leisure activities or where we want to live, whether it's near cities, mountains, plains or oceans, or even the kinds of people we want as friends.

The process of recovery is about growing and changing. Certain events in our lives can change the course or direction you thought you were going. Recovery is not only about regaining what you lost but about adjusting to the change. Recovering from a brain injury is kind of like reinventing yourself on some level. Not to say that you entirely lose your previous identity or self image, but your perspective of the world and of yourself may change

Another perspective of recovery is about returning to the familiar, to whom you were, to the friends and family that you knew and to a place of comfort. It's like "coming home." So where is home for you now? Where do you feel the most comfortable, happy and at peace? Is it the home of your childhood or is it the home you left before your brain injury?

You've heard the old saying, "Home is where the heart is." So where is this place? To some "coming home" isn't really a physical location. It is a place inside of you. It is a state of mind, as they say, or a state of being your true self. It is a place where you can make sense of the world and trust your gut feelings and your intuition. In order to achieve this state of being, it requires you to slow your life down and become more conscious. This allows time for introspection, to gain insight and the ability to make confident decisions and wise choices.

When you are feeling stronger, find ways to immerse yourself creatively through music, art, writing, reading, inspiring others, hobbies, etc. Find ways to give back to those caring people who have helped you in any way. As you heal and start to reach out and interact more, there may be a desire to bring meaning and purpose into your life. Also, there may be a yearning to have a sense of belonging — to be part of something or a group, a place where you feel validated, a place where you give and receive respect, love and support and above all joy, fun and laughter. Perhaps it is with your friends and co-workers, in your career, family, community, church, or in nature.

And finally, rather than focusing on your disabilities, focus on your abilities. When you shift your attention, you will be surprised to find new skills that you have acquired while learning to adjust and compensate to the changes. Take a moment now and honestly ask yourself, "What's new and different about me that I like?" "What's new and different about me that other people like?"

NO TIME LIMITS

Give yourself all the time you need to heal. Avoid putting yourself on a timetable. Your recovery is a major life transformation. Be prepared to change your life to work with your injury, not against it. Before launching into an activity, ask yourself, "Will this make me feel better?" Give yourself double the amount of time you would have previously given yourself to complete a task.

COMMENTS WE'VE ALL HEARD

Without a full understanding of the symptoms of MTBI, well-meaning people may say something that is meant to make you feel better, but it is not helpful because you might feel confusion or guilt for not being the person you used to be. Remember to forgive them for they mean well. Life is different now. Here are some comments we have heard:

- "You look fine."

- "You don't look sick."

- "Oh, that happens to me all the time."

- "That's just part of getting older."

- "So, just get a different job."

- "How much longer does this go on?"

- "You're still seeing doctors!?"

- "It could have been worse."

- "Just snap out of it."

THE HEALNG POWER OF HUMOR

Humor has long been known to heal the body and the spirit. Don't let the trauma of your injury prevent you from finding humor in life. Laughter has the power to heal and can make a big difference in your journey. When you are forced to deal with difficult people and situations, a little humor can go a long way. If you don't have a sense of humor, find one. It's impossible to underestimate the power of laughter.

SPECIAL DEVICES AND ACCESSORIES
TO PROMOTE HEALING

During the recovery process, it is important to use all means to make your life more comfortable. By taking some of the environmental stress off the brain it will expedite recovery.

The following list of adaptive devices can make your life easier:

- Special earplugs to filter out unwanted noise; ER15/25 noise-dampening ear filters; or noise-canceling headphones

- A dental mouth guard, or splint, to prevent damage to the teeth from clenching and grinding; these may be used during the day or at night

- Lenses and filters for glasses to protect sensitive eyes (sunglasses and visors inside of buildings)

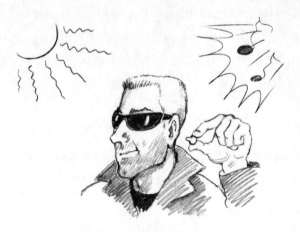

- Prism glasses to help when you are reading the computer screen

- Cushions to support the back and cervical spine

- Special pillows for sleeping

- Slant boards for use in reading

- Ergonomically correct chairs

- Watch, clock or cell phone alarms as reminders for medications and appointments

- Large, plain wall calendar

- Daily or weekly planner to keep track of appointments and necessary daily tasks

- Dry Erase boards placed around the house to share messages between family members and/or communication notebooks to write down messages and confirm plans with family members

- Icepacks for the neck or back

- Orthotics (special shoe inserts)

There are organizations that help returning veterans understand their rights, protect their interests, and ensure that they receive all benefits to which they are entitled.

CHAPTER 13

WHAT ARE
MY RIGHTS?

It is important to know that you have rights as a member of the military. Maneuvering through the medical and legal systems with a traumatic brain injury can be very difficult. If you, or a member of your family, are a "casualty" of war, you may qualify for benefits. The term "casualty" can refer to individuals who are injured, sick, hospitalized, or have been killed.

The administrative process that determines the rights of a veteran who suffers from TBI or PTSD can be complicated and lack advocacy on the veteran's behalf. Moreover, this process may decide the amount, if any, of disability benefits a discharged or separated veteran receives, or whether an injured veteran will be involuntarily separated.

If you are a veteran and lack guidance and information, this process can leave you significantly shortchanged. For example, a veteran whose MTBI or PTSD has resulted in an involuntary separation, may have in fact, been qualified to perform duties that would have allowed him or her to continue to serve. Therefore, veterans facing administrative procedures related to their injuries may want to retain counsel to protect their interests and ensure that they receive all benefits to which they are entitled.

An attorney can help you file claims and understand compensation ratings in the VA system. Furthermore, an attorney will argue on your behalf to ensure that you receive the outcome that your personal situation warrants.

There are organizations that help returning veterans, for example, Lawyers Serving Warriors. This organization provides legal representation to veterans of Operation Enduring Freedom (OEF) and Operation Iraqi Freedom (OIF) who have been referred into the disability evaluation system.

If you are a veteran who has already received a final determination related to your injury or disability, you are not without recourse. Lawyers Serving Warriors, which is

a project under the National Veterans
gram (NVLSP), can assist you in appea
award. More information is available a　　　　...vɔp.org/
Information/LSW/.

There are various proposals to increase funding for
evaluations and treatment of traumatic brain injuries
and other medical health issues. Surveys reveal that
one of the nation's top priorities is to provide medical
care to injured, sick, and disabled veterans. The military is responding to these needs by developing treatment centers.

Men and women returning home from the battlefield
should be welcomed home and recognized for their service. A new book by Elaine Gray Dumler, entitled The Road
Home: Smoothing the transition back from deployment,
supplies great information and resources for service
members facing deployment, reunion, and reintegration.
Operation Iraqi Freedom and the Soldier and Family Assistance Center also provide information to help military
members and their families find the correct resources for
their individual needs. You will find more organizations
listed in the Resources section in the back of this handbook.

Time saving tips and important things to remember for insurance and legal purposes:

- Collect copies of all medical documents, since you won't know what is important when contacting new medical providers or filing claims.

- Seek assistance, such as from the National Veterans Legal Service Program (NVLSP) or an attorney, as early in the process as possible.

- Write down the names, phone numbers, and dates of all contacts, and keep them in one place.

My Thoughts and Observations

You have just taken a detour on your life's journey.
There is so much more to experience and discover
if you are open to the endless possibilities.

CHAPTER 14

HEY, DO I GET MY OLD LIFE BACK?

Many of us ask, "When can I return to duty?" or, "When can I do the things that I used to do?" The honest answer is . . . who knows? You may find that you don't want your old life back. Maybe the stress and confusion of your old life are no longer desirable, or maybe you just aren't able to do what you used to do before the injury.

You have just taken a detour on your life's journey. There is so much more to experience and discover if you are open to the endless possibilities. Try new things but respect your new limitations. Remember not to force yourself. Discover what you enjoy doing now. Really, when you think about it, we are all growing and changing in many ways.

The core essence of who you are will never change; it is how you choose to express it from now on. You have just experienced a significant, life-changing event. It is your choice if you will be the victim or the victor. In the early stages of recovery, you may play both roles of victim and victor. Months or even years later, as you look back, you will be amazed at how far you have come in your recovery and in reinventing yourself.

Perhaps, you might view it as a second chance or the beginning of the next chapter in your life. Use this transition in a positive way. This will be one of the greatest challenges you will ever face and some of the greatest gifts that you will ever receive.

It is exciting to learn, as the latest research confirms, that we all have magnificent brains. In the next chapter, you will be encouraged by the landmark studies that reveal how the brain has the ability to heal and change in ways you never imagined.

IT'S NOT ABOUT YOU

When we have a life-altering event such as a brain injury, it is natural to take things more personally. It may seem that friends, work associates, and even loved ones do not understand. If they have not experienced a head injury, they may not have an understanding of what you are going through. No one can possibly know your personal journey in this recovery process.

Try to educate them by telling them what you are experiencing so that they can be as helpful as possible. It is difficult not to take things personally, particularly when you are overloaded, fatigued, and in pain. This may be a first-time experience for everyone involved. Seek out fellow veterans and organizations that give advice, assistance, and treatment. Join support groups, share experiences, and learn from others. Don't forget to share the humorous incidents because laughter is a powerful healer.

The Department of Defense, the Veterans Administration (VA), and other military organizations are increasing the diagnostic, treatment, and rehabilitative services to help the returning troops and veterans in their recovery and transition into civilian life. Thanks to caring individuals and to nonprofit organizations, newsletters, blogs and articles for raising the awareness of the plight of our injured warriors.

Seek out concerned people who want to make a difference. It's not just about you – it's about all of us. It's about

all of us taking part in recognizing the sacrifice the sur-
viving men and women, returning from military service,
made to protect our country. Many of them left their careers and loved ones behind including children. It is up to
all of us to understand the impact that MTBI and PTSD
have made on them and to find better ways to help them.
Employers need to understand that there is a valuable
human being behind those eyes that sincerely wants to
fulfill their hopes and be a benefit to society. It's about
all of us, including the injured, to be compassionate toward those who misunderstand and those that are mis-
understood.

My Thoughts and Observations

The human brain is an amazing and flexible organ.
This is one of the many reasons why the brain
can be rehabilitated following an injury.

CHAPTER 15

WHAT'S THE GOOD NEWS?

THE AMAZING BRAIN

The human brain is an amazing and flexible organ. It weighs about three pounds and contains approximately 100 billion nerve cells (Restak, 2001)[1]. It is believed that the 100 billion neurons in the brain are able to talk with each other through one or more links. Once a linkage is formed, it becomes stronger through repetition. This is one of the many reasons why the brain can be rehabilitated and retrained after it is injured.

Dr. Eric Braverman (2004), in his book *The Edge Effect*, states that the difference between a brain that is resourceful and functioning well and one that isn't is only 100 milliseconds of brain speed.[2] As the brain ages or be-

comes injured in an accident, it may process information more slowly. However, with practice and determination and by working to improve memory, speed of processing and focused concentration, you can overcome what you think is holding you back. At the same time, you may learn strategies to compensate. Some skills may be taken away or diminished, but you may also gain new skills that you never thought were possible.

WHAT IS BRAIN NEUROPLASTICITY?

Neuroplasticity is the brain's ability to change itself, it is trainable. When the brain is injured in an accident, such as a blast injury, car accident, or sports-related accident, it is believed that the brain can open old pathways or re-generate new pathways to help it function more normally again. Treatment to help the brain regain its skill is called cognitive retraining.

The brain has a left and right hemisphere and four major lobes – frontal, parietal, temporal, and occipital. The corpus callosum connects the two halves of the brain to each other. It is believed that different areas of the brain are dedicated to perform different functions. For example, the left hemisphere oversees linear functions and language, mathematical computation, reading, verbal memory,

word recall, etc. The right hemisphere has to do with such things as nonlinear, creative thinking, humor, simple math computation, musical talents,etc. The Frontal Lobe is very important in brain injury and controls reasoning, problem solving, and planning. The Parietal Lobe assists with orientation and sensory stimuli. The Occipital Lobe regulates visual reception and processing; and the Temporal Lobe controls auditory reception and language. Please refer to *Figure* 3 below:

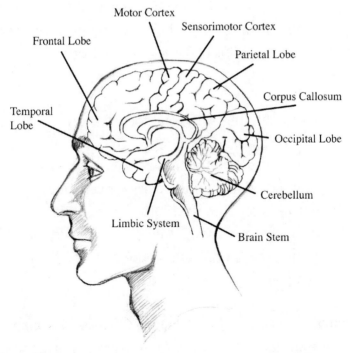

Figure 3

Recent research and the progress of of brain imaging studies are highlighting the fact that many functions occur in many areas of the brain. Through these sensitive diagnostic tools brain functions will be more clearly identified.

The good news is that the brain is highly resilient. This means that it can compensate for problems and/or it can be rehabilitated to perform more normally again, even following an injury. The brain has the ability to change with brain fitness exercises. If you would like to learn more about the magnificent brain, we highly recommend the book, *The Brain That Changes Itself*, by Norman Doidge, MD.[3]

It is important to talk with your doctor before initiating a program. The brain needs to rest initially following an injury before it begins retraining exercises. When you start exercising the brain, perform tasks for very brief periods of time (five to ten minutes). Discovering your tolerance level will allow you and your therapist to design your program around the specific amount of time and the type of tasks that you perform.

Change your activity by going for a walk, do breathing exercises, or dance to music. Do whatever it takes to in-

crease the blood flow to give your brain a boost in oxygen in a gentle way, especially in the beginning. You will be surprised how a ten or fifteen minute break can sharpen your thinking. You may need to rest and close your eyes for a period of time to recharge the brain. Then go back to the project or activity for brief periods, followed by relaxing and recharging breaks. Alternating brain rest and stimulation is called PACING. This is a very important activity to accelerate brain recovery.

When you are ready, here are some tips for TRAINING your brain:

1. Focus on NEW learning—play a musical instrument, learn to speak a new language, try new tasks and activities.

2. Start your brain training with tasks that you can accomplish without significant effort.

3. Use the idea of REVERSALS—e.g., use your left hand versus your right hand, perform visual versus auditory tasks, etc.

4. Engage in tasks that encourage the brain to become FLEXIBLE in its thinking patterns (e.g., say patterns like AB 1, 2; CD 3, 4; EF 5, 6, etc).

5. Stimulate the brain by listening to music and try

to recall the words. Read articles and try to recall one or two things that you read. Then, try to recall them an hour later.

6. Refer to the resources section for suggested reading.

Try not to get discouraged, especially if you find it hard in the beginning to concentrate or focus. A trained cognitive therapist will help you design a cognitive program that will improve your brain function at a pace that is best for you.

THE PATH OF MYSTERY

One of the great mysteries in life is "WHY" something happens. Why did I sustain an injury? Why am I in so much pain? Why is my loved one suffering so much? Unfortunately, we frequently don't get to know why something happens—we only know that we have a new opportunity in life to respond in a way that will advance our healing and strengthen our internal life force.

For those who have faith, this type of injury can be a call to faith. For those who don't, this can be a beckoning to something much bigger. We did a little study over time

with our clients who had suffered a brain injury. When they had completed their treatment, they were asked why they believed they had sustained this type of injury, if given the choice, would they move along this path and take this same journey again. Without exception, they said, "yes," they would, by choice, have the injury because it was a rich life experience; the majority of the individuals believed that it opened a door to a spiritual journey for them.

The mystery of life comes in many forms. Your nature will be tested and your true strengths will shine through. It is sometimes difficult to see the gifts of such a long and difficult journey with so little relief. Many believe that it builds patience and endurance, and others talk about the ability to find compassion for others through their own suffering.

Some individuals talk about learning to forgive another person or a situation. It is truly an opportunity to question all of your previous beliefs and listen to a deeper calling. Some believe that, when the whisper doesn't get your attention, you may be awakened by something more profound—like a brain injury, a physical loss, or an emotional trauma.

Although the road has many twists and turns, the learning experience is unique. It takes a great deal of strength and courage to believe that you will recover, to shed the bitterness and anger that you may feel for what may appear to be senseless suffering. By taking care of yourself and following a path of recovery, you give everyone hope. It is a precious gift to allow others to help you. Aspire to find hope and love in those around you. You are not alone.

MEDICAL DEFINITION
OF MTBI

The Mild Traumatic Brain Injury Committee of the Head Injury Interdisciplinary Special Interest Group of the American Congress of Rehabilitation Medicine published the following, which is a more specific medical definition of MTBI (1993):

A patient with mild traumatic brain injury is a person who has had a traumatically induced physiological disruption of brain function, as manifested by at least one of the following:

1. Any period or loss of consciousness

2. Any loss of memory for events immediately before or after the accident

3. Any alteration in mental state at the time of the accident— feeling dazed, disoriented, or confused

4. Focal neurological deficit(s) that may or may not be transient, but where the severity of the injury does not exceed the following:

  • Post-traumatic amnesia (PTA) not greater than twenty-four hours

  • After thirty minutes, an initial Glasgow Coma Scale (GCS) of 13 to 15*.

  • Loss of consciousness of approximately thirty minutes or less

* Glasgow Coma Scale (GCS) is a neurological scale with a 1 to 15 point scoring system that is used to record levels of consciousness. It assesses best eye response, best verbal response, and best motor response. The lowest GCS score possible is a sum of 3; and the highest is 15, "fully awake."

APPENDIX B

SYMPTOM QUESTIONNAIRE
FOR MTBI

The following questionnaire (which begins on the next page) was designed to evaluate many areas of cognitive functioning based on the perceptions of the individual. It is used to measure progress over time. It is a valid and reliable tool used to discriminate between mild to moderate TBI and non-injured individuals. It is suggested that you retake this Symptom Questionnaire every three to six months to measure your progress.

SYMPTOM QUESTIONNAIRE FOR MTBI

Name: _____

Date:_____

Please read this list (or it will be read to you) and indicate any problems that you may be having. Rate your problems on this scale: Almost Never, Occasionally, Sometimes, Frequently, Almost Always. Circle the category that best matches your response.

Memory

1. Are you losing or misplacing items?

Almost Never I Occasionally I Sometimes I Frequently I Almost Always

2. Are you forgetting what people tell you?

Almost Never I Occasionally I Sometimes I Frequently I Almost Always

3. Do you forget where you parked your car?

Almost Never I Occasionally I Sometimes I Frequently I Almost Always

4. Are you forgetting what you've read?

Almost Never I Occasionally I Sometimes I Frequently I Almost Always

5. Are you having difficulty remembering things from the past?

Almost Never I Occasionally I Sometimes I Frequently I Almost Always

Attention and Concentration

1. Are you having trouble concentrating?

Almost Never I Occasionally I Sometimes I Frequently I Almost Always

2. Do you have difficulty concentrating in noisy environments?

Almost Never I Occasionally I Sometimes I Frequently I Almost Always

3. Do you have difficulty concentrating on more than one thing at a time?

Almost Never I Occasionally I Sometimes I Frequently I Almost Always

4. Do you have difficulty focusing your attention while reading or watching TV?

Almost Never I Occasionally I Sometimes I Frequently I Almost Always

5. Are you having difficulty staying focused when you are driving?

Almost Never I Occasionally I Sometimes I Frequently I Almost Always

Language and Communication

1. Do you have difficulty understanding other people or following a conversation?

Almost Never | Occasionally | Sometimes | Frequently | Almost Always

2. Do you have difficulty thinking of words?

Almost Never | Occasionally | Sometimes | Frequently | Almost Always

3. Do you have problems expressing yourself in writing?

Almost Never | Occasionally | Sometimes | Frequently | Almost Always

4. Do you have difficulty expressing yourself verbally (e.g., do people ask you to repeat yourself)?

Almost Never | Occasionally | Sometimes | Frequently | Almost Always

5. Do you have difficulty spelling words?

Almost Never | Occasionally | Sometimes | Frequently | Almost Always

Balance/Coordination/Sensory Function

1. Do you find you have difficulty with handwriting, hitting a ball, riding a bicycle, or doing something that used to be easy to do?

Almost Never I Occasionally I Sometimes I Frequently I Almost Always

2. Do you have problems with balance or coordination?

Almost Never I Occasionally I Sometimes I Frequently I Almost Always

3. Do you experience increased fatigability?

Almost Never I Occasionally I Sometimes I Frequently I Almost Always

4. Do you experience loss or decrease in sense of taste?

Almost Never I Occasionally I Sometimes I Frequently I Almost Always

5. Do you experience loss or decrease in sense of smell?

Almost Never I Occasionally I Sometimes I Frequently I Almost Always

6. Do you experience physical pain?

Almost Never I Occasionally I Sometimes I Frequently I Almost Always

7. Do you experience sleep disturbance?

Almost Never I Occasionally I Sometimes I Frequently I Almost Always

Visual-Perception

---

1. Do you have increased sensitivity to light?

Almost Never | Occasionally | Sometimes | Frequently | Almost Always

2. Do objects seem closer or farther away than they actually are?

Almost Never | Occasionally | Sometimes | Frequently | Almost Always

3. When reading, do printed letters appear to change or change position? Do you see two of things when there is only one?

Almost Never | Occasionally | Sometimes | Frequently | Almost Always

4. Do you have difficulty focusing your eyes on objects?

Almost Never | Occasionally | Sometimes | Frequently | Almost Always

5. Do you feel dizzy or nauseous?

Almost Never | Occasionally | Sometimes | Frequently | Almost Always

---

Executive Function

1. **Do you have difficulty planning work or leisure activities?**

Almost Never | Occasionally | Sometimes | Frequently | Almost Always

2. **Do you have problems setting goals and priorities?**

Almost Never | Occasionally | Sometimes | Frequently | Almost Always

3. **Do you have difficulty starting new tasks?**

Almost Never | Occasionally | Sometimes | Frequently | Almost Always

4. **Do you have difficulty monitoring and correcting your errors?**

Almost Never | Occasionally | Sometimes | Frequently | Almost Always

5. **Do you have difficulty changing from one task to another?**

Almost Never | Occasionally | Sometimes | Frequently | Almost Always

Emotional Functioning

1. Have you noticed increased moodiness?

Almost Never | Occasionally | Sometimes | Frequently | Almost Always

2. Do you lose your temper more quickly than before?

Almost Never | Occasionally | Sometimes | Frequently | Almost Always

3. Do you feel depressed?

Almost Never | Occasionally | Sometimes | Frequently | Almost Always

4. Do you have feelings of anxiety or nervousness?

Almost Never | Occasionally | Sometimes | Frequently | Almost Always

5. Do family and friends comment on changes in your behavior?

Almost Never | Occasionally | Sometimes | Frequently | Almost Always

6. Do you have incresed irritability?

Almost Never | Occasionally | Sometimes | Frequently | Almost Always

Finances and Measurements

1. **Do you have difficulty performing simple addition and subtraction?**

Almost Never | Occasionally | Sometimes | Frequently | Almost Always

2. **Do you have difficulty making change at the store?**

Almost Never | Occasionally | Sometimes | Frequently | Almost Always

3. **Do you have difficulty balancing your checkbook as accurately as before?**

Almost Never | Occasionally | Sometimes | Frequently | Almost Always

4. **Do you have difficulty paying your bills on time?**

Almost Never | Occasionally | Sometimes | Frequently | Almost Always

5. **Do you have difficulty calculating the appropriate measurements for receipes or other projects?**

Almost Never | Occasionally | Sometimes | Frequently | Almost Always

Organization and Sequencing

1. Do you have difficulty following the steps of a recipe?

Almost Never I Occasionally I Sometimes I Frequently I Almost Always

2. Are you having difficulty attending to your mail on a regular basis?

Almost Never I Occasionally I Sometimes I Frequently I Almost Always

3. Are you having difficulty doing or keeping up with normal routine household chores?

Almost Never I Occasionally I Sometimes I Frequently I Almost Always

4. Do you have difficulty doing more than one thing at a time?

Almost Never I Occasionally I Sometimes I Frequently I Almost Always

5. Do you have difficulty effectively managing your time?

Almost Never I Occasionally I Sometimes I Frequently I Almost Always

Safety

1. Do you forget to turn off the iron, stove, or other electrical appliances?

Almost Never I Occasionally I Sometimes I Frequently I Almost Always

2. Do you forget where you're going when you get into your car?

Almost Never I Occasionally I Sometimes I Frequently I Almost Always

3. Do you forget to lock your doors at home?

Almost Never I Occasionally I Sometimes I Frequently I Almost Always

4. Do you forget important appointments (e.g., picking up your children, etc.)?

Almost Never I Occasionally I Sometimes I Frequently I Almost Always

5. Do you feel that your awareness levels are less than they should be?

Almost Never I Occasionally I Sometimes I Frequently I Almost Always

UNDERSTANDING YOUR RESULTS

There are 53 items on the Symptom Questionnaire for MTBI. By adding up the number of each response (Almost Never, Occasionally, Sometimes, Frequently, and Almost Always), and dividing each one by the total number of items in the questionnaire (53), you will get a percentage of how often you have symptoms at each severity level. For example, if you have 10 in the Almost Always category and divide 10 by 53, your result will be 19%. You can re-take the functional symptom questionnaire over time to measure your progress.

APPENDIX C

MEDICATION RECORD

Date Started	Medication Name	Dosage and Directions	Comments

APPENDIX D

RECORD OF HEALTH CARE

PROFESSIONALS

Doctor/Provider Name	Address	Telephone Number

ENDNOTES AND REFERENCES

We have chosen to document references to studies that are quoted in the text to make it easier for the reader. These references that are presented in chronological order by chapters are extensive enough to expand your knowledge of relevant information.

Chapter 1

1. Signature Injury of the current war. The Associated Press, April 9, 2009, MSNBC.com. Returning troops tested for brain injuries.
2. MTBI has affected more than 300,000 military service personnel. Hoge, C.W., H.M. Goldberg, and C.A. Cisno. 2009. Care of War Veterans with Mild Traumatic Brain Injury—Flawed Perspectives. *New England Journal of Medicine* 360(16): 1588-1591.
3. Studies being done at Johns Hopkins reveal that even if you were not hit in the head or knocked out, the indirect powerful pressure waves caused by a bomb may affect the brain: Hagerman, E. 2008. Blast trauma. E. *Popular Science* 49-53.

4. The history of mild traumatic brain injury has been documented for more than a century. During the 1860's, Doctor John Erichsen in London, talked of "obscure injuries of the nervous system" that happened as a result of railway collisions. He believed that damage to the spinal cord and brain caused "nervous shock to the system." Erichsen, JE. 1882, On concussion of the spine. In Nervous Shock and Other Obscure Injuries of the Nervous System and their Clinical Medical and Legal Aspects. London: Longmans, Green and Company.

5. The symptoms of mild brain injury are much more serious than previously believed or shown through testing. Russell Packard writes, "The sequelae of even minor head injuries may reflect a more severe disturbance of brain function than investigative techniques can document." Packard, R.C. 1993. Mild head injury. *Headache Quarterly* 4(1): 42-52.

6. Approximately 1.4 million people sustain a brain injury in the United States each year, and 800,000 of those are believed to be "mild traumatic brain injuries." More recent studies of individuals returning from combat in Iraq and Afghanistan reveal that at least 59% of those who were exposed to a blast were diagnosed with TBI (traumatic brain injury) ; 56% of those were considered to be moderate or severe; and 44% were mild. Okie, S. 2005. Traumatic Brain Injury in the War Zone. *The New England Journal of Medicine* 35(20): 2043 – 2047.

7. Survivors of TBI are particularly susceptible to major depression, generalized anxiety disorder, and post-traumatic stress disorder. Russoniello, C., M. Fish, J. Parks, J. Rhodes, B. Stover, et. al. 2009. Training for optimal performance biofeedback program: A cooperative program between East Carolina University and the United States Marine Corps Wounded Warrior Battalion East. *Biofeedback* 37(1):12-17.

Chapter 2

1. The correlation between high altitude and headaches has been well documented. Serrano-Duenas, M. 2005. High altitude headache. A prospective study of it's clinical characteristics. Cephalgia 25(12):1110-1116 and Queiroz, L.P. A. Rapoport, 2007. High altitude headaches. *Current Pain and Headache Reports* 11(4).

2. When changes in barometric pressure occur, individuals with MTBI complain of headaches intensifying, especially when storms move in and the barometer drops. Some countries are on the cutting edge of weather-based health forecasts that alert people to barometric pressure changes. For example, Germany and Canada have on-line services. For more information about this service, click on www.ec.gc.ca/Envirozine.

Chapter 3

1. The Mayo Clinic developed a technique called canalith repositioning (1994), where the head is maneuvered in various positions to help eliminate the dizziness. This is accomplished by moving the calcium crystals in the inner ear. *Mayo Clinic Health Letter* December, 1994. 12(12).

Chapter 7

1. Pets are good medicine http://www.Petside.com. Singer, J. March, 2009 Freedom Dogs improve returning soldier's lives. http://www.FreedomDogs.org

Chapter 9

1. It has been said that "there should be no need for a bottom line here. The use of these drugs in an already disrupted physiological system will further induce neurological and cognitive decline. They should be avoided in survivors of MTBI." Jay, G. 2000. *Minor Traumatic Brain Injury Handbook: Diagnosis and Treatment.* New York: CRC Press.

Chapter 10

1. ....states that physical exercise can sharpen your thinking, improve memory skills, and prepare the brain for learning. He also talks about the many scientifically proven benefits of aerobic exercise and emphasizes the relationship of exercise and mood elevation. Ratey, J. and E. Hagerman. 2008. **Spark: The Revolutionary New Science of Exercise and the Brain.** New York: Little, Brown and Company.

Chapter 11

1. Biofeedback/neurofeedback is an important treatment technique that has been used in the VA system to assist recovering veterans. Peniston, E. G. and P.J. Kulkosky. 1991. Alpha-Theta Brainwave Neurofeedback Therapy for Vietnam Veterans with Combat-Related Post-Traumatic Stress Disorder. *Medical Psychotherapy, An International Journal* 4: 47-60. and Peniston, E. G., D. A. Marion, W. A., Deming. 1993. EEG Alpha-Theta Brainwave Synchronization in Vietnam Veterans with Combat Related Post Traumatic Stress Disorder and Alcohol Abuse. *Medical Psychotherapy, An International Journal* 6: 37-50

2. These modalities have also been identified as being successful in the treatment of MTBI (Ayers, M., 1987). Electroencephalographic Neurofeedback and Closed Head Injury, Head Injury Frontier, National Head Injury Foundation Annual Conference 380-392, Bounias, M., R. G.Laibow, A. Bonaly, et. al. 2001. EEG Neurofeedback Treatment of Patients with Brain Injury, Part 1: Typographical Clarification of Clinical Syndroms. *Journal of Neurotherapy* 5(4): 23-44 and Thornton, K. 2000. Improvements/Rehabilitation of Memory Functioning with Neurotherapy/QEEG Biofeedback. *Journal of Head Trauma Rehabiliation* 15(6): 1285-1296.

3. Currently, there are numerous biofeedback and neurofeedback training programs for optimal performance that have shown good preliminary results in reducing or eliminating symptoms of TBI

and PTSD Russoniello, C., M. Fish, J. Parks, et. al. 2009. Training for optimal performance biofeedback program: A cooperative program between East Carolina University and the United States Marine Corps Wounded Warrior Battalion East. *Biofeedback* 37(1):12-17.
4. Proactive methods to help troops develop a resiliency to combat stress are being implemented and studied. Pyne, J. and R. Gevirtz. 2009. Psychophysiologic assessment and combat post traumatic stress disorder. *Biofeedback* 37(1): 18-23.

Chapter 15
1. The brain weighs about 3 pounds and contains 100 billion nerve cells. Restak, R. 2001. *Mozart's Brain and the Fighter Pilot.* New York: Harmony Press
2. *The Edge Effect* states that the difference between a brain that is resourceful and functioning well and one that isn't is only 100 milliseconds of brain speed. As the brain ages or becomes injured in an accident, it may process information more slowly: Braverman, E. 2004. *The Edge Effect.* New York: Sterling Publishing Company, Inc.
3. The brain has the ability to change with brain fitness exercises. If you would like to learn more about the magnificent brain, we highly recommend *The Brain That Changes Itself* by N. Doidge, New York: Viking, 2007.

RESOURCES

RECOMMENDED MILITARY WEB SITES

www.OneFreedom.org
ONE Freedom offers programs that teach veterans and family members vital information about the brain and body, how they are changed by stress, and, through a powerful framework, educate how to maintain balance and strengthen resilience and understanding. Call 303-444-1221 or 888-334-VETS (8387).

www.CoalitionForVeterans.org
The Coalition for Iraq and Afghanistan Veterans (CIAV) is a national, nonpartisan partnership of organizations committed to working with and on behalf of all military, veterans, families, survivors, and providers to strengthen the existing system of care and support for all those who have been affected by the wars in Iraq and Afghanistan. Among the many opportunities to heal, they provide Return to Work (R2W), which is a nonprofit organization with free services to newly disabled Americans, including injured soldiers. Unlike a traditional employment agency, R2W offers unique online services with the personal touch of counselors who truly care about wounded warriors.

www.WoundedWarriorResourceCenter.com

The Wounded Warrior Resource Center (WWRC) Web site is a Department of Defense Web site that provides wounded service members, their families, and caregivers with information they need on military facilities, health-care services, and benefits. It supports access to the Wounded Warrior Resource Call Center and trained specialists who are available twenty-four hours a day, seven days a week by phone at 1-800-342-9647, or by e-mail at wwrc@militaryonesource.com.

http://www.militaryhomefront.dod.mil/operationwarfighter

MilitaryHOMEFRONT is the Department of Defense Web site for official Military Community and Family Policy (MC&FP) program information, policy, and guidance designed to help troops and their families, leaders, and service providers. Whether you live the military lifestyle or support those who do, you'll find what you need.

http://lawyersservingwarriors.com/

Lawyers Serving Warriors is a project of the National Veterans Legal Services Program. As the voice of veterans' rights for the last twenty-five years, the National Veterans Legal Services Program (NVLSP) works to ensure that the U.S. government keeps its pact with our nation's 25 million veterans. NVLSP is an independent, nonprofit veterans service organization that has assisted veterans and their advocates since 1980. Call 202-265-8305.

www.swords-to-plowshares.org

Swords to Plowshares Iraq Veteran Project ensures that recent veterans receive the support, services, and protection they need to successfully transition home. GWOT veterans are eligible for free legal representation for VA claims and military discharge reviews, as well as for employment and training, transitional housing, social services, and benefits counseling. Services are available to all GWOT veterans, former active duty, guard, and reserve, with any type of discharge. Swords to Plowshares Iraq Veteran Project is located in the San Francisco area, call 415-252-4788.

www.vets4vets.us
Vets4Vets is a nonpartisan veterans' peer-support organization dedicated to helping Iraq and Afghanistan veterans heal from any negative aspects of service and war. Vets4Vets pays ALL expenses for OIF/OEF vets to fly to weekend peer-support workshops. Call 520-319-5500. Veterans of Foreign Wars Foundation.

www.vfwfoundation.org
The VFW Foundation is committed to improving the lives of veterans and service personnel, their families, and the communities in which they live and work through a variety of programs. Their programs include free long-distance communication for troops, free financial grants for military members and families in need, and free assistance with VA claims. Call 816-756-3390.

www.woundedwarriorproject.org
WWP's Project Odyssey aims to teach coping skills for combating post-traumatic stress. Jacksonville, FL, 904-296-7350.

www.vba.va.gov/
Vocational rehabilitation and veterans benefits information.

www.tricare.mil/cap
Assistive technology and accommodations information.

www.veteransgreenjobs.org
Veterans Green Jobs provides exemplary green jobs education and career development opportunities for military veterans, empowering

and supporting them to lead America's transition to energy inde-
pendence, ecological restoration, community renewal, and economic
prosperity.

www.jan.wvu.edu
Job Accommodations Network (JAN).

www.va.gov
Department of Veterans Affairs (VA).

www.dodvets.com
DoD Disabled Veterans.

www.myhealthevet.va.gov
Interactive VA personal health site.

www.dvbic.org
The Defense and Veterans Brain Injury Center.
The mission of the Defense and Veterans Brain Injury Center (DVBIC)
is to serve active duty military, their dependents and veterans with
traumatic brain injury (TBI) through state-of-the-art medical care, in-
novative clinical research initiatives and educational programs.

www.ninds.nih.gov/disorders/tbi/tbi.htm
The National Institute of Neurological Disorders and Stroke.

www.bobwoodrufffamilyfund.org/about_brain_injury.shtml
Bob Woodruff Family Fund for Traumatic Brain Injury.

www.EEG4veterans.com
Web site for free Neurofeedback for veterans.

RECOMMENDED HEAD INJURY WEB SITES

www.biausa.org
Brain Injury Association of America can direct you to local offices in your area. Search their web site for other resources including location of Neuropractitioners in your area.

www.biacolorado.org
Brain Injury Association of Colorado.

www.headinjury.com
This is a nonprofit organization with an abundance of information to build skills and to participate in discussion groups. You can also link to resources, rehab, and research sites for all types of head injuries.

www.eeginfo.com
A Web site with information about neurofeedback.

www.emdr.com
Learn about eye movement desensitization and reprocessing (EMDR). It has been proven to produce profound treatment effects in eliminating or greatly diminishing the emotional distress related to a traumatic memory. Clients who experience the EMDR processing also gain important cognitive insights.

www.health.mil/dcoe.aspx

Defense Centers of Excellence for Psychological Health and Traumatic Brain Injury.

www.ASHA.org
The American speech-Language Hearing Association maintains this Web site to help you locate Cognitive Therapists and speech/Language Pathologists in your area.

www.traumahealing.com
Learn about Somatic Experiencing® which is a body-awareness approach to trauma being taught throughout the world. It is the result
of over forty years of observation, research, and hands-on development by Dr. Peter Levine. SE® restores self-regulation, and returns a
sense of aliveness, relaxation and wholeness to traumatized individuals who have had these precious gifts taken away. Peter has applied
his work to combat veterans, rape survivors, Holocaust survivors,
auto accident and post-surgical trauma patients, chronic pain suf-
ferers, and even to infants after suffering traumatic births.

www.PuppiesBehindBars.com
This is a program that trains inmates to raise puppies to become
service dogs for the disabled. The dogs give unconditional love to
the inmate trainers and the bond that is created with wounded veterans returning from Iraq and Afghanistan is life changing.

The following Web sites are used to improve cognitive functioning:
> **www.puzzlersparadise.com**
> **www.CogniFit.com**
> **www.braingle.com**
> **www.Lumosity.com**

RECOMMENDED BOOKS

Brain Injury Survival Kit: 365 Tips, Tools & Tricks to Deal with Cognitive Function Loss, by Cheryl Sullivan. New York: Demo Medical Publishing, 2008.

Change Your Brain, Change Your Life, by Daniel G. Amen, New York: Three Rivers Press, 1998.

Healing Trauma: A Pioneering Program for Restoring the Wisdom of Your Body, by Peter A. Levine, PhD. Louisville: Sounds True, 2008.

I'll Carry the Fork: Recovering a Life After Brain Injury, by Kara L. Swanson. Scotts Valley: Rising Star Press, 1999.

Mild Traumatic Brain Injury: A Clinician's Guide: Edited by Michael J. Raymond, Thomas L. Bennett, Laurence C. Hartlage and C. Munro Cullum. Pro-ed Publishers, Austin, Texas, 1999.

My Stroke of Insight: A Brain Scientist's Personal Journey, by Jill Bolte Taylor, PhD. New York: Viking Penguin, 2008.

Recovering from Traumatic Brain Injury is a pamphlet provided by the Defense and Veterans Brain Injury Center, which is the primary operational TBI component of the Defense Centers of Excellence. All service members should be aware of the valuable information and resources packed into this small and easy to read pamphlet. Call 800-361-4653 or click on www.quickseries.com.

Spark: The Revolutionary New Science of Exercise and the Brain, by John J. Ratey, MD. New York: Little, Brown and Company, 2008.

Tears of a Warrior: A Family's Story of Combat and Living with PTSD, by Janet J. Seahorn, PhD, and E. Anthony Seahorn, MBA. Ft. Collins: Team Pursuits, 2008.

The Body Bears the Burden: Trauma, Dissociation, and Disease, by Robert C. Scaer, MD, PhD. Binghamton: Da Capo Press, 2998.

The Brain That Changes Itself, by Norman Doidge, MD. New York: Viking Penguin, 2007.

The Evaluation and Treatment of Mild Traumatic Brain Injury, edited by Nils R. Varney and Ricard J. Roberts. Lawrence Enbaum Associates Publishers, Mahwah, New Jersey, 1999.

The Road Home: Smoothing the Transition Back from Deployment, by Elaine Gray Dumler. Frankly Speaking, 2009.

Walking the Tiger: Healing Trauma; the Innate Capacity to Transform Overwhelming Experiences, by Peter A Levine and Ann Frederick. Berkeley: North Atlantic Books, 1997.

ABOUT THE
AUTHORS

MARY ANN KEATLEY, PhD, CCC, is a speech-language patholo-gist and neurotherapist who has specialized in the treat-ment of traumatic brain in-juries and other neurological conditions for more than 30 years. Her broad experience includes neurorehabilitation, 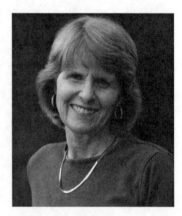 research, and publications in the fields of speech-language pathology, rehabilitation, and outcomes. She is a Profes-sional Speaker and gives presentations and training in the field of brain injuries and has a private practice in Boulder, Colorado. She is the co-founder of the Brain Injury Hope Foundation.

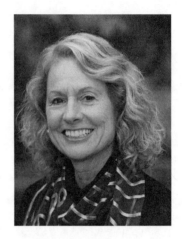

LAURA L. WHITTEMORE has been in the field of psychology and education and an entrepreneur for more than 30 years. She sustained a TBI in 2001, caused by a horseback riding accident. Fortunately, she was wearing a helmet. Since her life-changing, wake up call, she has focused her gifts gained through her recovery process into writing, speaking, life coaching, and creating memory fitness programs. She is on the board of the Brain Injury Hope Foundation. Laura has two children and six grandchildren and lives, hikes, and skis in sunny Colorado.

HOW TO ORDER

Online Orders: www.BrainInjuryHopeFoundation.org
Telephone Orders: 303-484-2126
Email Contact: sales@BrainInjuryHopeFoundation.org

Recovering from Mild Traumatic Brain Injury (MTBI)..............$12.95
A Handbook of Hope for Our Military Warriors
and their Families

Sales Tax: Please add 4% for books shipped to Colorado addresses.

Shipping: Please add $3.50 for the first book and $1.50 for each
additional book. Please call or email for shipping rates for
quantities of books over 5.

Ask for Quantity Discounts starting at 25 books.

Proceeds from book sales are donated to the
Brain Injury Hope Foundation.
P.O. Box 1319
Boulder, CO 80306